Atlas of Practical Applications of Cardiovascular Magnetic Resonance

Developments in Cardiovascular Medicine

Previous volumes are still available

Atlas of Practical Applications of Cardiovascular Magnetic Resonance

edited by

Guillem Pons-Lladó, M.D.
Director, Cardiac Imaging Unit
Cardiology Department
Hospital de la Santa Creu I Sant Pau
Universitat Autónoma de Barcelona
Barcelona, Spain

Francesc Carreras, M.D.
Cardiac Imaging Unit
Cardiology Department
Hospital de la Santa Creu I Sant Pau
Universitat Autónoma de Barcelona
Barcelona, Spain

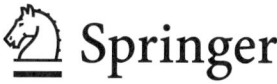 Springer

Guillem Pons-Lladó, M.D.
Director, Cardiac Imaging Unit
Cardiology Department
Hospital de la Santa Creu I Sant Pau
Universitat Autónoma de Barcelona
Barcelona, Spain

Francesc Carreras, M.D.
Cardiac Imaging Unit
Cardiology Department
Hospital de la Santa Creu I Sant Pau
Universitat Autónoma de Barcelona
Barcelona, Spain

Library of Congress Cataloging-in-Publication Data

Atlas of practical applications of cardiovascular magnetic resonance / edited by Guillem
    Pons-Lladó and Francesc Carreras
        p. ; cm. – (Developments in cardiovascular medicine ; 255)
    Includes bibliographical references and index.
    ISBN 0-387-23632-5 (alk. paper)   e-ISBN 0-387-23634-1
      1. Heart—Magnetic resonance imaging—Atlases. I. Pons- Lladó, Guillem, 1951- II.
    Carreras, Francesc. III. Developments in cardiovascular medicine ; v. 255.
      [DNLM: 1. Cardiovascular Diseases—diagnosis—Atlases. 2. Magnetic Resonance
    Imaging—methods—Atlases. WG 17 A8843947 2005]
    RC670.5.M33A85 2005
    616.1'207548—dc22

                                                                    2004059144

Printed in the United States of America.

9 8 7 6 5 4 3 2

springer.com

Contents

Chapter 3: *Acquired Diseases of the Aorta*

Guillem Pons-Lladó

Chapter 4: *Study of Valvular Heart Disease*

Luís J. Jiménez Borreguero

Chapter 5: *Cardiovascular Magnetic Resonance of Ischemic Heart Disease*

Sandra Pujadas, Francesc Carreras

Chapter 6: *Cardiac and Paracardiac Masses*
Francesc Carreras

Chapter 7: *Diseases of the Pericardium*
Guillem Pons-Lladó

Chapter 8: *Congenital Heart Disease*
Maite Subirana, Xavier Borrás

Xavier Borrás, MD. Cardiac Imaging Unit. Cardiology Department, Hospital de la Santa Creu i Sant Pau, Associate Professor of Medicine, Universitat Autónoma de Barcelona. Barcelona, Spain.

Francesc Carreras, MD. Cardiac Imaging Unit. Cardiology Department, Hospital de la Santa Creu i Sant Pau, Universitat Autónoma de Barcelona. Barcelona, Spain.

Luís J. Jiménez-Borreguero, MD. Cardiology Department. Hospital Príncipe de Asturias, Alcalá de Henares, Madrid, Spain.

Guillem Pons-Lladó, MD. Director, Cardiac Imaging Unit. Cardiology Department, Hospital de la Santa Creu i Sant Pau, Universitat Autónoma de Barcelona. Barcelona, Spain.

Sandra Pujadas, MD. Cardiac Imaging Unit. Cardiology Department, Hospital de la Santa Creu i Sant Pau, Universitat Autónoma de Barcelona. Barcelona, Spain.

Maite Subirana, MD. Director, Unit of Congenital Heart Diseases. Cardiology Department, Hospital de la Sant Creu i Sant Pau, Universitat Autónoma de Barcelona, Barcelona, Spain.

Oliver M. Weber, PhD. Department of Radiology, University of California, San Francisco, California, USA.

List of Contributors

Six years have passed since the edition of our Atlas of Practical Cardiac Applications of MRI. Fortunately, the technique has experienced during this time a continuous development that demanded a new updated version of the book. One of the consequences of this growing process has been the adoption of the term Cardiovascular Magnetic Resonance (CMR) to refer to the technique, and this is why the title of the present version of the book has changed slightly in relation to the first one.

Merits of CMR were evident from its beginning, early in the eighties. There was a time, however, when CMR ran the risk of becoming a luxury diagnostic tool, either confined to the experimental field or limited to serve as an occasional resource for selected clinical entities, only applied by even more selected specialists. Things have changed, for the benefit of cardiology, during the last few years, particularly since CMR has proved to be a very useful technique also in the study of ischemic heart disease, which constitutes the main issue of concern in cardiology today. As a consequence, CMR is starting to play a relevant role in clinical practice, and it has become an issue of interest for the educated cardiologist. Evidence for this is the increasing body of research articles which, on CMR in myocardial infarction, for instance, has more than doubled since 1999 compared with the five-year previous period, or the publication of major textbooks on CMR, up to three in the last two years. Also, there is a strong academical interest on the technique, with a growing number of specialized meetings and activities from associations aimed to spread knowledge on the technique, as the Society for Cardiovascular Magnetic Resonance, or the Working Group on CMR of the European Society of Cardiology.

Updated sources of information are thus needed for clinicians interested in the field and, particularly, for those demanding to be initiated in it. The present version of this Atlas is intended to be one of these sources. Most of the authors are clinical cardiologists devoted to the field of cardiac imaging who have the privilege of being experienced in those techniques that are ultimately useful on the clinical problems they are dealing with. During the last 25 years, we have learnt, as every cardiologist involved in cardiac imaging has done, that the actual value of a technique lies in its ability to give reliable answers to relevant clinical questions. When such a technique is, in addition, unique in doing that, then it becomes essential. Echocardiography has fulfilled these requirements in many aspects for many years, and its role is not disputed. CMR is gaining the same respect also in a good deal of issues, and today is no longer an auxiliary tool but a first line method in many instances. The important point is to learn which ones. We hope that the examples presented in this book will help clinicians to learn *when* a CMR exam is useful and, also, *how* to plan and read CMR studies in every particular case.

The emergence of radiological techniques, like CMR or computed tomography, in the field of diagnostic cardiology, has raised the question of which specialist should be in charge of these studies. The technical complexity of CMR, and the wide variety of pulse sequences and acquisition strategies, made reasonable the direct participation of radiological teams. On the other hand, the even more complex spectrum of cardiovascular disorders and, particularly, the different clinical relevance of some of their aspects, seem to demand a cardiological view. In practice, excellent teams performing CMR may be found among radiologists specialized in cardiovascular diseases and, also, among cardiologists devoted to imaging, a close cooperation between them being the optimal approach. In our case, we have always agreed with our radiologist colleagues on the collaborative nature of this task. We are in debt to them, and we feel mandatory a mention of the radiology departments where the studies illustrating this book have been obtained:

- Radiology Department (Dr. Jordi Ruscalleda), Hospital de Santa Creu i Sant Pau, Barcelona, Spain.
- Corachán Magnetic Resonance Center (Dr. Carlos Alexander), Clínica Corachán, Barcelona, Spain.
- Balearic Magnetic Resonance Center (Dr. Darío Taboada), Clínica Femenía, Palma de Mallorca, Balearic Islands, Spain.
- Clinica Ruber and Hospital Ruber Internacional, Madrid, Spain

Guillem Pons-Lladó
Cardiac Imaging Unit
Department of Cardiology
Hospital de Santa Creu i Sant Pau
Barcelona, Spain

Glossary

Axial plane: horizontal transverse plane.

Black Blood Imaging: MR sequence in which blood does not generate signal, such as spin-echo sequences.

Breath-hold: voluntary interruption of the respiration necessary for the correct acquisition of fast sequences.

Cine MR: series of gradient-echo images obtained in consecutive phases of the cardiac cycle and displayed in a continuous loop sequence.

Coil: element of the MR system that generates the radiofrequency pulses used to excite the study subject (transmitting antenna), or that also receives the echoed pulses returned by tissues (receiving antenna). The same coil can act as both transmitter and receiver, or there can be two independent coils, one for each function.

Contrast: The difference in signal intensity between tissues in an image.

Contrast agent: A substance administrated to the patient in order to change the contrast between tissues (gadolinium-based contrast agents are used in clinical practice).

Coronal plane: vertical frontal plane.

Delayed contrast-enhanced imaging: CMR method that, by using Inversion-Recovery sequences, allows the identification of myocardial scar tissue due to the persistence of the contrast agent in areas of myocardial fibrosis up to 30 minutes after its administration, while it is washed-out from the normal myocardium, this resulting in a high signal intensity of the scarred tissue.

Echo planar imaging (EPI): technique enabling the obtention of an image by means of a single radiofrequency excitation in a time on the order of milliseconds.

Echo time (TE): time interval between the radiofrequency pulse emission excitation and the reception of the radiofrequency signal emitted by the tissues.

Fast low-angle shot: gradient-echo sequence that uses short repetition times and reduced matrix, thus allowing the acquisition of images in less than a second.

Fast SE sequence: A multiple echo spin-echo sequence which allows the acquisition of several lines of k-space within a repetition time.

Field strength: degree of intensity of the magnetic field generated by the system magnet (measured in Tesla units).

Field of view (FOV): dimension of the study window.

Flip angle: value reached by the precession angle when stimulated by a specific radiofrequency pulse.

Free induction decay (FID): name given to the radiofrequency signal emitted by the protons of tissue during relaxation after having been submitted to radiofrequency excitation at resonance frequency in the presence of an intense, external magnetic field.

Frequency encoding: a process which enables the location of a point along one of the axes of the study plane: along with phase encoding, it defines the position of this point in the study plane.

Gadolinium (chelated): paramagnetic contrast agent of intravascular and extracellular distribution that produces a change in T1 and T2 relaxation times of the tissues this improving their contrast in the images.

Gating: coupling between slice acquisition of a sequence and any cyclical physiological signal: ECG; respiration, peripheral pulse.

Gradient echo (GE): MR technique by which adequately contrasted images are obtained of dynamic structures and of blood flow. Due to the short repetition times employed, it is possible to include various excitations in one cardiac cycle time, which enables the obtention of dynamic cine MR sequences.

Interslice gap: distance, which does not appear in the image, that separates contiguous slices of a sequence.

Inversion Recovery sequence: MR sequence in which, by applying a 180: inversion RF pre-pulse, signal intensity and contrast between tissues is modified.

Inversion time: Time interval between the inversion pre-pulse and the acquisition of the echo in an Inversion-Recovery sequence.

K-space: Numerical matrix containing the information needed to produce an image. The Fourier transform (mathematical method) of k-space results in an image.

Magnetic resonance angiography (MRA): Contrast-enhanced MR technique that provides a 3D imaging of the vessels.

Matrix: number of information units (voxels) that constitute the image.

Multi-phase: any sequence in which each slice is obtained in multiple phases of the cardiac cycle.

Multi-slice: any sequence in which multiple contiguous slices are obtained during one acquisition.

Oblique plane: plane with a certain degree of angulation over any one of the standard planes (axial, coronal or sagittal).

Parallel imaging: Imaging technique that allows reconstruction of an image in less than the time required for conventional imaging by using the spatial information related to the different coils of the receiver array.

Phase encoding: a process which enables the location of a point along one of the axes of the study plane: along with frequency encoding, it defines the position of this point in the study plane.

Pixel size: dimensions (in mm) of the information unit in the two-dimensional representation of the image on the screen. Image resolution depends on pixel size, which varies according to field of view and matrix.

Precession angle: angle between the vector axis of the external magnetic field and the rotation axis of the hydrogen proton.

Pulse sequence: series of consecutive excitations and receptions, its analysis resulting in the acquisition of images with any one of the MR techniques.

Radiofrequency: fragment of the electromagnetic spectrum that includes waves with frequencies under 10^{12}. The radiofrequency waves used in MR have frequencies of 10 to 100 MHz.

Radiofrequency pulse: brief radiofrequency signal emitted to excite the protons of the hydrogen atoms of the study subject.

Relaxation time: time required for the returning to a resting state of the hydrogen protons after a radiofrequency pulse excitation. Longitudinal relaxation or T1 is the time it takes them to return to the basal precession angle. Transversal relaxation time or T2 is the time elapsed until the energy acquired by phase coherence, in which protons are under the influence of an external radiofrequency pulse, is lost.

Repetition time (TR): interval between the emission of two radiofrequency pulses.

Sagittal plane: vertical antero-posterior plane.

Scout image: initial planes of rapid acquisition used to locate the next sequences.

Segmented-K-space: fast imaging technique based on the obtention of grouped lines of information (segments) instead of the line-by-line method used in conventional techniques, this reducing the acquisition time of an image to a matter of seconds.

Signal void: area of absent signal due to the flow characteristics in a specific region of the slice plane: it appears in instances of high flow rate or of turbulence in gradient-echo sequences.

Signal averaging or number of excitations (NEX): number of repeat measurements required for a sequence to be obtained with adequate definition of the images.

Signal-to-noise ratio (SNR): relation between the signal intensity from tissue structures and the background image noise, upon which image quality depends.

Single phase: any sequence in which one or various slices are obtained, each one in a different phase of the cardiac cycle.

Single slice: any sequence in which the images are obtained from a single slice.

Slice thickness: width of the slice.

Slice: section of the study subject which is imaged.

Spatial resolution: ability to discriminate between two different structures in the image, depending on the field of view and the matrix size.

Spectroscopy: technique that permits the acquisition, in an area of a specific tissue displayed in the MR image, of the spectrum of concentrations of an element (usually phosphorus) according to the different chemical compounds in which it is present.

Spin echo (SE): MR sequence that provides images of adequate contrast between tissues and blood flow, as no signal is elicited by rapidly moving structures.

Steady state free precession imaging (SSFP): GRE sequence that provides faster acquisition times with a higher contrast between tissues than conventional sequences.

Tagging: MR technique in which equidistant crossing lines are magnetically preselected in the ventricular myocardium, allowing to track dynamic myocardial wall changes during the cardiac cycle.

Tesla: standard unit of magnetic field strength.

T1-weighted image: MR image in which the signal intensity of the tissues is predominantly dependent on T1.

T2-weighted image: MR image in which the signal intensity of the tissues is predominantly dependent on T2.

Ultrafast sequences: techniques applying information acquisition strategies designed to reduce the total time spent in the process of imaging.

Velocity-encoded MR imaging: MR sequence which permits flow measurements through a particular vessel by providing both, the area and mean velocities of the blood flow, of the vessel studied.

Voxel: tridimensional unit of the MR matrix that integrates the two dimensions constituting the pixel with the thickness of the slice.

Wash-out effect: effect by which the blood flowing in a direction perpendicular to the slice plane produces a characteristic absence of signal (signal void), in the spin-echo technique, due to the fact that the excited blood leaves the slice plane well before the echo signal is read.

Basics of Cardiac Magnetic Resonance and Normal Views

1

SANDRA PUJADAS
OLIVER WEBER

1.1 Definition and historical background

Magnetic Resonance (MR) is a physical phenomenon consisting on the emission of a radiofrequency (RF) signal by certain nuclei with an angular momentum (spin), such as hydrogen (^{1}H, proton), carbon (^{13}C), or phosphorus (^{31}P), after having been stimulated by RF pulses while being under the influence of an external magnetic field (B0). This phenomenon is based on the principle that these nuclei can absorb energy at a specific frequency, known as *Larmor frequency*.

Clinical MR imaging is based on the detection of hydrogen nuclei, which are widely present in all structures from the body in the form of water (H_2O) and fat. The physical phenomenon of nuclear MR was discovered in 1946[1]. The first clinical images obtained by this technique were published in 1973[2]. The evolution of computer technology in the 1980's allowed the development of first commercial equipments, with most applications focusing on the brain. Some early reports of cardiac applications were published in 1983[3]. Since then, cardiovascular MR (CMR) has experienced a continuous expansion[4,5] as is demonstrated by the amount of clinical reports on its applications, including reports from expert committees summarizing the present indications of the technique[6]. Currently, CMR is the newest and most complex of the cardiovascular imaging modalities, with diverse clinical applications spanning nearly every aspect of disease affecting the heart and blood vessels[7]. Noteworthy, 2003's Nobel prize in Physiology or Medicine was awarded to Paul Lauterbur and Peter Mansfield, who were recognized for their contributions to the basis for the development of magnetic resonance into a useful imaging method in the early 1970s.

1.2 Physical basis

Nuclei with a spin, exposed to an external magnetic field, act like magnetic dipoles. Magnetic dipoles under the influence of an external magnetic field (B0) do not align in a strictly static position. Instead, they exhibit an oscillation around their own axis parallel to the magnetic field (*precession* movement or *spinning*) (Figure 1.1). The dipol's deviation from the axis of the external field is called the angle of precession. Hydrogen nuclei have only two possible orientations in a magnetic field: parallel (low energy) or anti-parallel (high energy) (Figure 1.2).

The precession frequency of these nuclei is called Larmor frequency. It is proportional to the external magnetic field, with the proportionality factor γ usually given in units of MHz/T. For protons, $\gamma = 42.6$ MHz/Tesla, resulting in a Larmor frequency of 63.9 MHz at 1.5 T, a typical field strength in clinical MRI.

1.2.1 MR signal: Free Induction Decay

In the presence of an exterior B0 field, a slightly higher number of spins have a z-component parallel to B0 (z-axis) as compared to anti-parallel. This polarization is called net-magnetization. However, since the spins are oriented randomly with respect to the other two axes (x- and y-axis), the integral magnetization is parallel to B0. Therefore no precession occurs and no signal is detectable (Figure 1.3). When protons under the influence of an external magnetic field receive an energetic impulse by means of a RF wave pulse emitted at its resonance frequency, a deviation of the angle of precession is produced in the xy plane (flip angle) (Figure 1.4). Flip angle depends on the amplitude and duration of the RF pulse. On the other hand, the RF pulse induces all protons to precess in-phase, resulting in phase coherence. When the RF signal is interrupted protons are in phase. This oscillation can be detected by external receiver coils and results in a signal known as FID (Free Induction Decay) (Figure 1.5). However, the phase coherence will decay over time, and the spins will progressively and individually return to their basal state. The detection of this RF wave by a receiving coil constitutes the base for both the technique of MR imaging as well as for MR spectroscopy.

1.2.2 Relaxation

The return of the hydrogen nucleus to the basal state following the cessation of the RF pulse is called relaxation. Magnetization has vectorial characteristics and can be considered as constituted by a longitudinal component, parallel to the axis of the external magnetic field (z-axis), and by a transversal component orthogonal to it (xy-plane). The time constant, at which the longitudinal vector returns to its value prior to stimulation by the RF pulse is called longitudinal relaxation time, or T1. Recovery occurs exponentially as shown in a graph of signal intensity against time in Figure 1.6 (A). T1 depends on the tissue and on the external field strength. Typical values of T1 of biological tissue are in the order of a few hundred ms to a few seconds under field strengths available for clinical applications (Table 1.1). Longitudinal relaxation time depends on the molecular enviroment: T1 tends to be long in solids and short in mobile liquids. Differences in T1 between different tissues are partly responsible for MRI contrast between tissues.

The transversal vector (in the xy-plane perpendicular to the axis of the external magnetic field) reflects the energy secondary to the coherence in the spin phase of the different protons. In the absence of RF stimulation, each hydrogen nucleus spins with a different phase. The resultant net value is thus zero. When an RF pulse is applied, the nuclei couple in a phase (all spinning together at the same time) and the transversal vector is then maximal. After the RF signal has been switched off, the coherence and, thus, the energy contained in it dissipates. The loss of energy due to dephasing coherence is known as transversal relaxation. It occurs as an exponential decay with a time constant T2 (Figure 1.6 B). Transversal relaxation is conditioned by two factors: first, due to physical inhomogeneities in the local magnetic field, known as $T2^*$; and, second, by tissue composition (spin-spin interaction): T2. $T2^*$ is a much faster process than T2, but its effect can be reversed by applying a second RF signal pulse with a phase shift of $180°$. This procedure eliminates the nonvariable components while retaining only the influence of the tissue composition in the signal. Transversal relaxation time is very sensitive to the presence and type of other atoms that surround hydrogen originating the resonance signal. Therefore, it varies greatly according to the different tissues, but it is practically unaffected by the intensity of the external magnetic field. Typical values

FIGURE 1.1

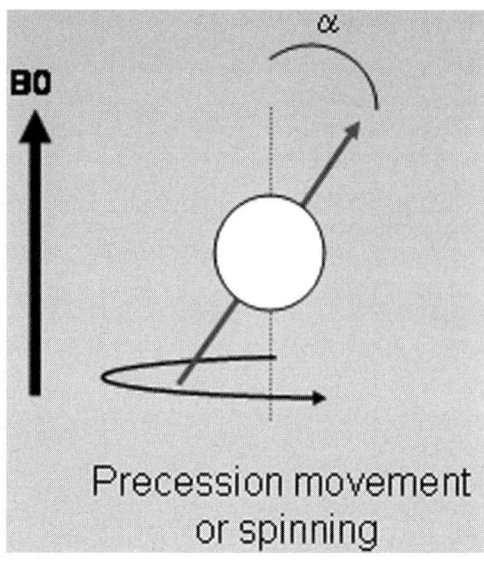

Precession movement or spinning

FIGURE 1.2

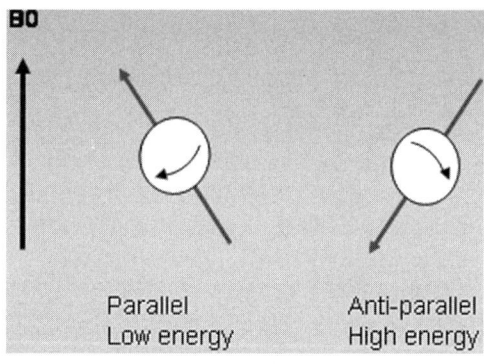

Parallel
Low energy

Anti-parallel
High energy

FIGURE 1.3

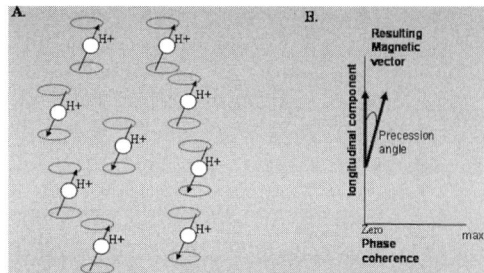

FIGURE 1.4

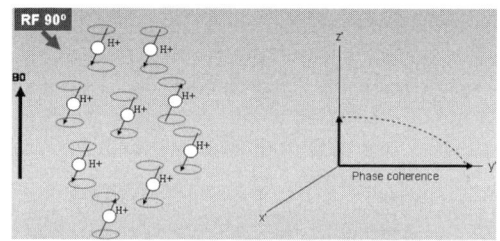

FIGURE 1.5

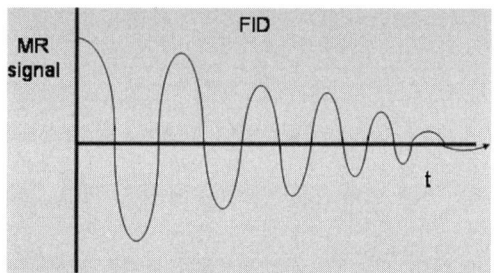

FIGURE 1.6

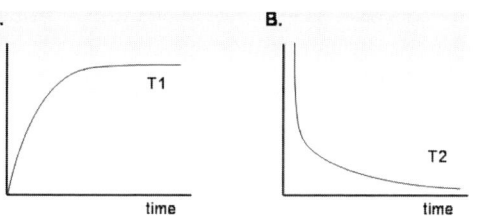

Table 1.1 T1 values at 1.5T[24]

Tissue	T1 (ms)
Blood	1200
Myocardium	880
Muscle	880
Lung	820
Fat	260

for T2 of biological tissues are in the range 20–200 ms.

Fluids are characterized by long T2 and T1, as opposed to macromolecules, which have short T2 and T1.

1.2.3 RF pulse and MR imaging

Signal intensity, and thus contrast in MR images, depend on proton density within the voxel (defining the maximal signal intensity available), as well as the relaxation parameters T1 and T2. Different pulse sequences emphasise contrast based on different specific parameters. For instance, T1-weigthed, T2-weighted, and proton density-weighted imaging sequences are available. Pulse sequences consist of a series of excitation/relaxation cycles. Most often, many cycles of excitation and relaxation are necessary in order to obtain the data for an entire image. The interval between two of these cycles is called repetition time (TR). The relative signal intensity of different tissues, which we call contrast, can be affected by varying the TR and the time between the RF pulse emission and signal reception (echo time, TE).

Images based on T1 relaxation time (T1-weighted) are obtained by means of short TR and TE. A short TR maximizes the effect of T1; a short TE minimizes the effect of T2. When imaging the heart this causes surrounding fat to appear with a high signal intensity (bright), the pulmonary air and the blood which flows rapidly to appear relatively dark, and the cardiac muscle to show an intermediate intensity. In order to enhance tissues with long T2 (T2-weighted images), much longer TR and TE must be used. A long TE enhances T2 contrast, and a long TR minimizes T1-contrast. This may constitute a limitation in the analysis of cardiac structures due to their rapid constant movement, which causes that images obtained with long TR and TE are highly affected by artefacts. Images obtained with long TR and short TE will show signal intensities mainly based on proton density, and with limited effects from T1 or T2.

1.3 Pulse sequences

Several MR techniques are useful for cardiovascular purposes (Table 1.2). Each technique provides particular information on different aspects of the cardiovascular system.

1.3.1 Classic Sequences

1.3.1.1 Spin-Echo

After a 90° pulse, protons initially precess in unison before rapidly dephasing due to both spin–spin relaxation (T2) and local field inhomogeneity (T2*). A 90° pulse, followed by a 180° RF pulse to refocuse the spins at TE/2, will lead to a signal peak at time point TE, called a spin echo (Figure 1.7). The effect of the

---

F. 1.1. Precession movement of spins in a magnetic field.
α, precession angle.

F. 1.2. Spins in a magnetic field (B0) have two orientations: parallel, in which precession movement has the same direction as the magnetic field; antiparallel, spinning in the opposite direction and, thus, possessing a higher energy.

F. 1.3. Hydrogen atoms under the influence of a strong external magnetic field. The magnetic dipoles are aligned with the external magnetic field, most of them in the same direction (parallel) and some in the opposite one (antiparallel) (A). The difference between both directions causes the resulting magnetic vector diverging from the direction of the vector of the external magnetic field with the precession angle. The hydrogen atoms spin in different phase, the value of phase coherence being thus null (B).

F. 1.4. Application of a RF pulse at resonance frequency of sufficient energy to increase the precession angle to 90° (90° pulse). Most of the magnetic dipoles orient themselves in an antiparallel direction. It can also be observed how the increase in the precession angle reduces the value of the longitudinal component of the resulting vector. The coherence phase value reaches its maximum as the majority of the atoms spin at the same time.

F. 1.5. Immediately after RF pulse is interrupted the magnetization precesses around the axis of the main magnetic field, and the spins will gradually dephase. As a result an RF signal is detected, though it rapidly decays.
FID, free induction decay; t, time

F. 1.6. **A.** Graph showing longitudinal magnetization returning exponentially to equilibrium (T1-relaxation). **B.** Tranverse relaxation (T2-relaxation) due to protons dephasing.

Table 1.2 Technical modalities of MRI and their applications in cardiovascular studies

Technique	Information	Application
SE, FSE	Static tomography	Morphology
GE, SSFP	Static/Dynamic tomography	Morphology/Function
MRA	Static tomography/3D view	Angiography
Velocity mapping	Flow curves	Flow/valvular studies
Myocardial tagging	Myocardial mechanics	Myocardial function
EPI	Static/Dynamic tomography	Perfusion studies
Spectroscopy	Chemical tissue composition	Metabolic studies

EPI, echo-planar imaging; FSE, fast spin echo; GE, gradient-echo; MRA, MR angiography; SE, spin-echo; SSFP, steady state free precession

180° pulse is to reverse the relative phase of the spins. Therefore, magnetic field inhomogeneities, which previously caused dephasing, now cause the spins to rephase. The resulting images are static, single-phase images, showing fat as high signal (bright) and myocardium as intermediate signal. Blood flowing orthogonal to the imaging slice appears dark because spins that have been excited by the 90° RF pulse have flown out of the imaging slice and do not experience the 180° refocusing pulse; they do thus not generate signal ("black blood" imaging). Stationary and slowly moving blood on the other hand appears bright thanks to its long T2 (Figure 1.8). When necessary, a pre-pulse can be applied to null the signal produced by the fat, a method known as fat-saturation.

In CMR, Spin-echo (SE) imaging is mainly used for morphological studies. It allows T1–weigthed or T2-weighted imaging with high spatial resolution and high signal-to-noise ratio (SNR). However, it is a relatively slow imaging technique (several minutes for a typical image). A faster variant of it is the turbo spin-echo sequence, discussed in paragraph I.3.2.1.

1.3.1.2 Gradient-Echo
In this type of sequence, no 180° pulse is applied. Instead, a bipolar gradient is used to generate a detectable echo (Figure 1.9). The proton dephasing, which is amplified by the magnetic gradient present during slice-selective excitation, is reversed by applying an equal but inverted gradient. Rephasing spins then generate the MR signal. The use of gradients rather than a RF pulse for echo formation allows to obtain the signal at very short TEs and TR; image acquisition can thus be significantly shorter than for spin echo

sequences[8]. To prevent magnetization from completely being saturated due to insufficient T1-relaxation, a lower flip angle (<90°) can be used (FLASH, fast low angle snap shot).

Multi-phase images, that may be displayed as cine-loops, can be obtained with this sequence (Figure 1.10 and Cine Loop 1.01 on CD). An additional property of this sequence is the visualization of blood turbulence as a "signal void" due to an increased phase incoherence in these areas[9] (Figure 1.11 and Cine Loops 2.04 and 3.01 on CD).

1.3.1.3 Velocity-encoded (phase contrast) MR imaging
This sequence is used for MR flow measurements. The technique is based on the principle that spins moving along a magnetic field gradient acquire a phase shift in comparison to stationary spins. The phase shift is proportional to the velocity of the moving spin. A phase (velocity mapping) and a magnitude (anatomy) image are generated simultaneously (Figure 1.12a and Cine Loop 1.02 on CD). Mean velocities values are obtained by this method. Therefore, by tracing the area of interest (Figure 1.12b) instantaneous flow values can be calculated as: area x velocity[10] (Figure 1.13). The velocity encoding (VENC) given by the operator defines the strength of the velocity-encoding gradients and determines the highest and lowest velocity encoded by a phase-contrast sequence. Therefore, VENC = 200 cm/s describes a measurable range of flow velocities of ±200 cm/s.

Phase-contrast provides a mean velocity obtained from averaging all measured velocities over a range of cardiac cycles with an overall error in flow measurement below 10%[11].

FIGURE 1.7

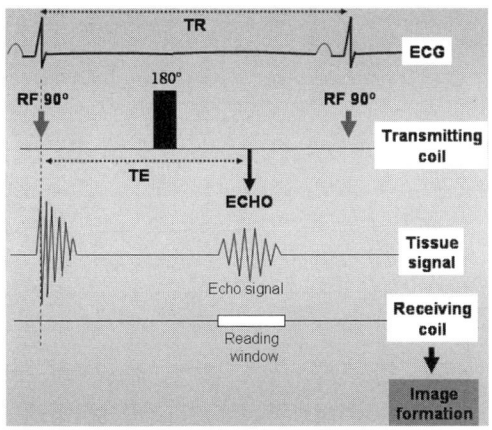

FIGURE 1.8

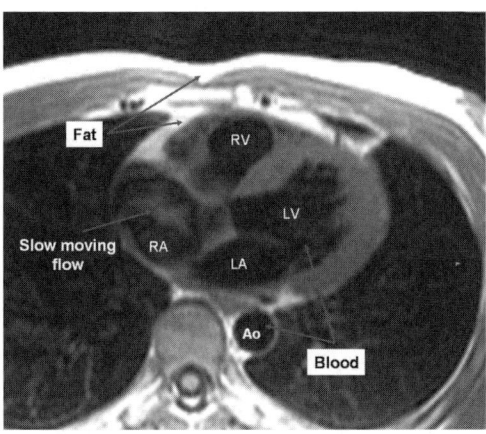

FIGURE 1.9

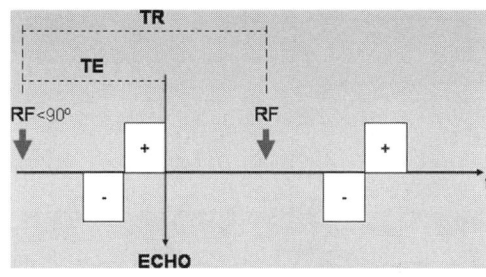

F. 1.7. Excitation sequence in the formation of a spin-echo image. Gated with the R wave of the ECG, a 90° RF pulse is emitted which generates a tissue response signal (not read). At the TE/2 time, a refocusing pulse of 180° is emitted. At a TE interval after the 90° RF pulse a tissue signal (echo) is produced, which is read by the receiving antenna for processing and image formation.
ECG, electrocardiogram; RF, radiofrequency; TE, echo time; TR, repetition time

F. 1.8. Spin-echo T1w image in a transverse plane showing the characteristic signal absence of moving blood in the cardiac chambers and vessels, as well as the high signal intensity generated by fat tissue. Myocardium shows an intermediate signal intensity. Notice that slow moving flow in the right atrium shows some signal that might lead to misinterpretation. These erratic signals of intraluminal flow may appear in cases of stasis or abnormally slow circulation.
Ao, aorta; LA, left atrium; LV, left ventricle; RA, right atrium; RV, right ventricle

F. 1.9. Gradient echo (GE) sequence. A bipolar gradient, instead of a 180° pulse, is inserted. The negative gradient (−) increases spin dephasing, while the positive lobe (+) refocuses the spins resulting in a signal peak. Echo times with GE sequence are shorter than with SE imaging, allowing faster image acquisition.
RF, radio-frequency pulse; TE, echo time; TR, repetition time; t, time

It has to be noted that peak velocities with this method might be underestimated due to factors such as angle effects in case of eccentric jets (slice not being orthogonal to the flow jet) or low temporal resolution.

Sources of error:

(a) *Mismatch of VENC*: The better the VENC matches the real velocity of the region of interest, the more precise the measurement becomes[11].

• VENC too high: **Noise** in velocity images increase with larger VENC values affecting mainly peak velocity determination (which can be masked by noise peaks).

• VENC too low: Setting the encoding velocity below the peak velocity in the vessel of interest results in **aliasing**. It can be easily perceived in the velocity

images, in which voxels of presumed peak velocity have an inverted signal intensity compared with that of surrounding voxels, resulting in a characteristical "black and white" appeareance.

(b) Imaging plane should be positioned orthogonal to the direction of the flow and *through-plane* flow encoding used. This is a multiphase sequence, a set of 16 frames per cardiac cycle is considered to be sufficient for typical heart rates. Lower temporal resolution leads to flow and peak velocity underestimation.

FIGURE 1.10

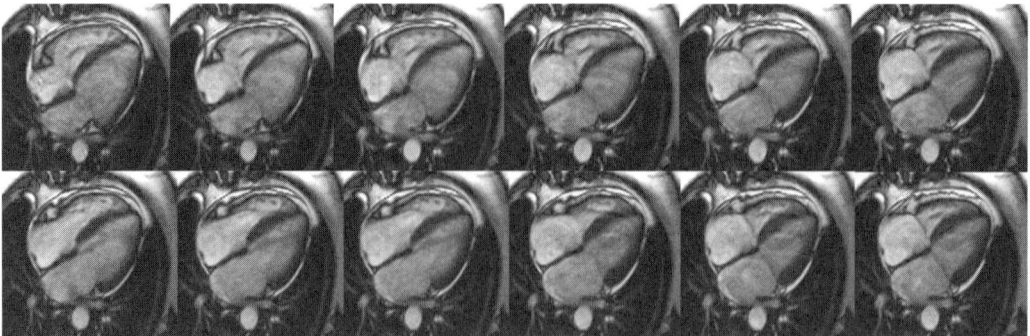

FIGURE 1.11

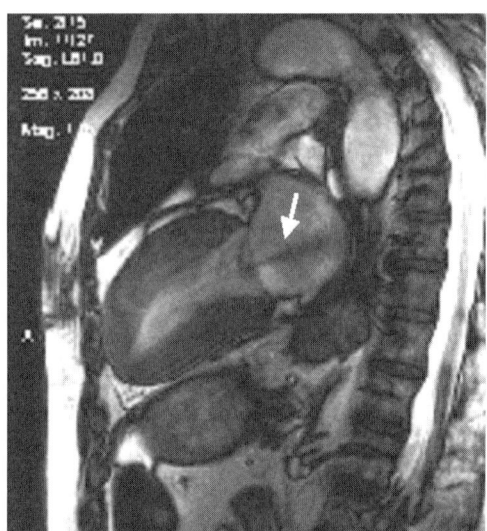

FIGURE 1.12

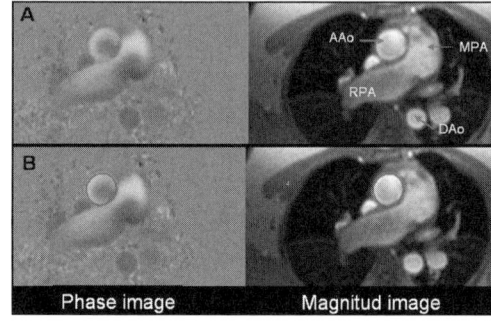

FIGURE 1.13

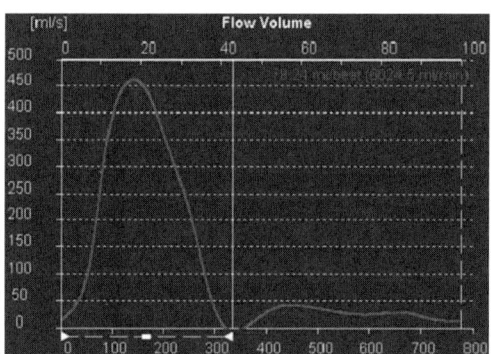

F. 1.10.   Multiphase GE sequence. Twelve frames showing different phases of the cardiac cycle in a left ventricular horizontal long-axis view (4 chamber). These images are usually displayed as a loop. LA, left atrium; LV, left ventricle; RA, right atrium; RV, right ventricle

F. 1.11.   SSFP sequence on a longitudinal vertical plane of the left ventricle showing a signal void (arrow) indicating turbulent flow due to mitral regurgitation.

F. 1.12.   Ascending aorta velocity-encoded MR imaging. Axial plane at the level of great vessel. On the left the phase image and on the right the corresponding magnitude image. By tracing the area of interest (B) flow values can be calculated.
AAo, ascending aorta; DAo, descending aorta; MPA, main pulmonary artery; RPA, right pulmonary artery

F. 1.13.   Graph of flow volume measurement derived from phase velocity mapping sequence shown in Figure 1.12

FIGURE 1.14

FIGURE 1.15

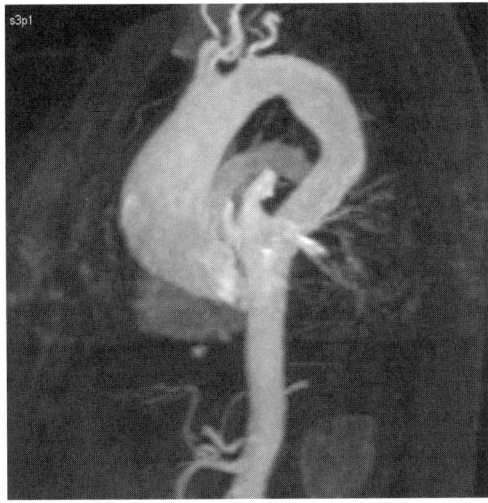

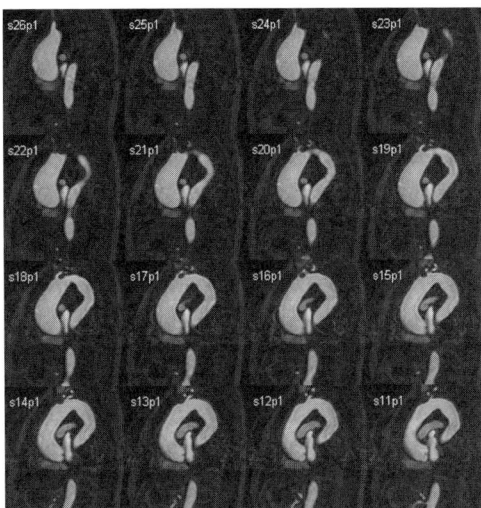

F. 1.14.   Angiogram of the aorta in a patient with an aneurysm of the ascending aorta.

F. 1.15.   Set of dynamic images used to create a MIP.

1.3.1.4 MR Angiography

A combination of T1-shortening contrast agent and fast T1 weighted imaging methods allows the acquisition of an entire three-dimensional high-resolution volume data set in a single breath-hold. After the contrast injection, the agent will rapidly circulate through the vascular territory, being in the arterial phase for a short interval of time[12]. It is important to time the MR data acquisition so that it coincides with the period of peak signal in the vessel of interest. Appropriate timing can be achieved with different approaches:

- Test bolus: A small amount of contrast is injected (2 ml of gadolinium-based) and a rapid imaging sequence is applied covering the region of interest. By this method we obtain a determination of the time interval between injection and peak enhancement in the region of interest. The MRA study is then performed based on the previously determined time delay between contrast injection and peak signal.
- Automatic bolus track: An initial low resolution sampling sequence is obtained while injecting the contrast. When signal enhancement increases above a preset threshold, this initial sequence is terminated and the MR study is begun. It can also be activated manually so that at the moment we see the region of interest enhancing we start the MRA acquisition.

Based on a set of maximal-intensity projection (MIP) images, an angiogram is created (Figure 1.14). However, it should be noted that MIPs can generate some artefacts that may lead to erroneous results. Therefore, it is always preferable to review the base images in order to achieve a correct interpretation of the study (Figure 1.15).

Paramagnetic contrast (e.g., Gadolinium-based) is injected intravenously with a power injector at 2–3 ml/s. Image data are collected as the contrast agent flows through the vascular territory of interest, depicting the blood vessels by means of a high signal intensity. This sequence is mainly used for vascular studies.

1.3.2 New Modalities

1.3.2.1 Fast Spin Echo o Turbo Spin Echo

As discussed above, the spin echo sequence is a relatively slow imaging technique. It can be accelerated by acquiring several echoes after a single excitation[13]. After the first 90° a series of multiple 180°-pulses are generated, obtaining for each one a spin echo with a different phase-encoding gradient (echo train), thus allowing the acquisition of multiple lines of k-space (see k-space) within a given TR. The number of echoes used within a TR is called Echo Train

Length (ETL) or Turbo Factor (TF). A higher ETL will decrease the acquisition time, but may result in noticeable image blurring due to T2-effects for high ETL-values.

1.3.2.2 Fast gradient-echo and steady state free precesion (SSFP)

Based on strategies of reducing TR and TE parameters, a category of techniques known as fast GE (turboFLASH, GRASS, SPGR) allow an image to be obtained in less than 1 second[14] and can be implemented on conventional systems. By combining these fast gradient-echo sequences with a segmented k-space acquisition method, in which all the data that correspond to an image is acquired in the form of portions (segments), high-resolution cine images can be obtained in one breathhold[15].

More recently, the development of steady-state free precession (SSFP) MRI techniques (known as *balanced fast-field echo* in Philips, *true-FISP* in Siemens, *FIESTA* in General Electric) have shortened significantly the acquisition time (by a factor of 2 to 3) at similar temporal and spatial resolutions due to the very short repetition times achievable. Additionally, the (SNR) and the contrast-to-noise (CNR) ratio of SSFP have been shown to be substantially higher compared with conventional techniques[16,17] (Figure 1.10 and Cine Loop 1.01 on CD). It has thus found wide-spread use for the imaging of cardiac function, and other applications are constantly being explored. However, this sequence is very sensitive to susceptibility artefacts such as in metallic prosthetic valve. Magnetic field homogeneity (shimming) optimization is therefore crucial.

Additionally, further reduction of the scan time or improvement in spatial resolution can be achieved by using parallel imaging techniques such as (SENSE) in Philips, IPAT in Siemens, or ASSET in General Electric[18].

1.3.2.3 Inversion-Recovery and Saturation-Recovery

By applying a pre-pulse at the start of the sequence and acquiring the echo at a chosen delay time (inversion or saturation recovery time), signal intensity and contrast between tissues can be modified.

IR sequences are used for viability studies (see Chapter 5). Paramagnetic contrast such as gadolinium-DTPA reduces T1 relaxation time. By applying a $180°$ RF pulse and acquiring the echo at an appropriate time delay (inversion time), normal myocardial signal is nulled whereas myocardium with contrast retained is shown as "bright" (high signal due to its shorter T1)[19] (Figure 1.16).

For SR sequences a $90°$ RF pulse is used. Thus, SR results in less contrast differences but faster acquisition. They are thus a good alternative for first-pass perfusion studies[20].

1.3.2.4 Echo-Planar Imaging (EPI)

This sequence provides an extremely fast acquisition time using very fast switching bipolar gradients that allow the filling of all the k-space lines after a single RF pulse[21]. However, spatial resolution is very poor. It is mainly used in perfusion studies as a hybrid sequence EPI/Turbo Field Echo (TFE).

1.4 Image formation

1.4.1 Slice selection

One of the main advantages of CMR is the possibility of obtaining true 2D-slices or 3D-data sets in any spatial orientation. In order to produce a selective excitation of a plane a magnetic gradient along its orthogonal direction is generated. Thus, a different magnetic field will be perceived by spins in different regions and so, these spins will precess at a different frequency. By setting the frequency of the RF pulse to the resonance frequency of the desired location, only spins in this slice fulfil the resonance frequency and experience the RF pulse. Spins outside the slice are not excited and thus do not generate detectable signal.

1.4.2 Image reconstruction

After initial slice selection, additional gradients are applied in orthogonal directions to encode for spatial information: *phase-encoding and frequency-encoding*. The scan duration is a function of TR and the total number of excitations required to acquire all the k-space lines (phase-encoding steps). The number of k-lines to be filled is defined by the matrix size, rectangular field of view, number of averages, etc.

1.4.2.1 Frequency-encode direction (read out gradient)

A magnetic gradient within the slice plane forces spins located in different columns to

FIGURE 1.16

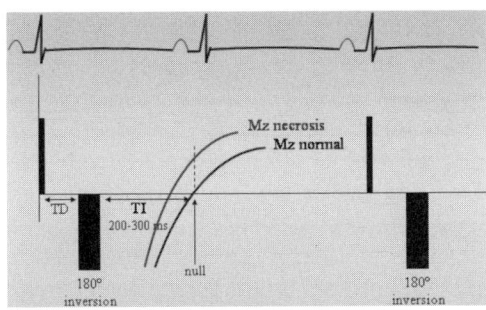

FIGURE 1.17

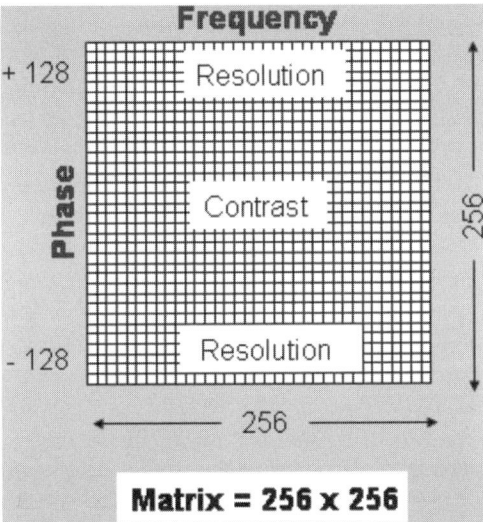

FIGURE 1.18

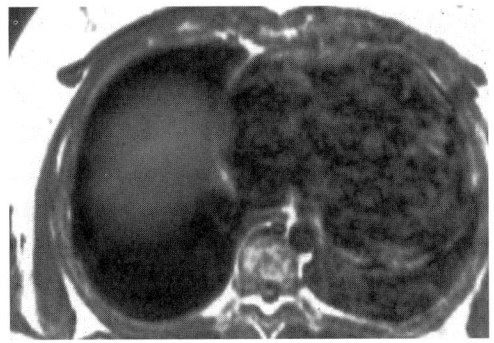

F. 1.16. Diagram for the segmented inversion recovery turbo-FLASH sequence with inversion time set to null normal myocardium after the administration of contrast agent. Contrast is retained in infarct areas shortening T1. Consequently, when normal myocardial signal is null, these infarcted areas show a bright signal due to its shorter T1 (see chapter 5 for details). TD, trigger delay; TI, inversion time. Adapted from (19)

F. 1.17. K-space diagram for an acquisition matrix of 256 × 256. The x and y axes represent the frequency- and phase-encode directions, respectively. The time interval between two acquired lines (phase-encode direction) corresponds to the TR of the sequence. A complete line of k-space (frequency-encode direction) is acquired during the readout. The scan duration is a function of the repetition time and the total number of k-space lines (phase-encode).

F. 1.18. Example of a poor quality SE image caused by signal artifacts due to poor ECG syncronization.

precess at a different frequency. Frequencies can be analysed and separated by means of their signal amplitude (Fourier transformation), resulting in a single projection in the frequency direction. The amplitude obtained for each frequency is the result of the sum of all the spins in that column.

1.4.2.2 Phase-encode direction

Just before the signal acquisition, a magnetic gradient parallel to the slice plane and orthogonal to the frequency encoding direction is applied. This gradient will temporarily change the frequency of precession of the spins. The amount of accumulated phase difference will depend on the spin position through the column. Different phase-encoding gradients encode for different lines in the k-space.

1.4.3 K-space

The set of raw data obtained from each different echo constitutes what is known as k-space or Fourier space. Thus, k-space is a numerical matrix containing the information needed to produce an image, each point in k-space providing information about the entire image. Points near the centre of k-space (low frequency-encoding regions) determine the general appearance and contrast of the image, whereas peripheral points (high frequency-encoding regions) account for image edge detail (Figure 1.17).

1.5 Study Methodology and potential problems

The main difficulty for imaging the heart is that it is a moving structure itself, and it is also affected by respiratory motion. These motion components potentially causing blurring in the images when not properly accounted for (Figure 1.18). It is essential in any case to synchronize MR acquisition to the ECG: since the formation of an MR image typically results from a series of consecutive acquisitions, an accurate timing of these excitations with respect to the cardiac cycle is mandatory in order to freeze the cardiac motion and obtain a final image of an adequate quality.

In order to minimize artefacts produced by respiratory movements there are two different methods: a) Patient breath-hold, which is the most commonly used as it is easy to perform; new sequences have considerably shortened acquisition times, and consequently breath-holding times; b) Respiratory synchronization techniques such as navigator that, however, considerably prolongs study time, which makes their use less desirable in clinical routine.

1.5.1 Technical equipment

- A high field strength magnet with in the range of 0.5 to 3.0 Tesla. Current work-horse for CMR is a 1.5 T magnet strength, which allows application of the latest sequences to perform perfusion and viability studies. There is a trend towards higher field strength (3.0 T) mainly in neurological applications, but also in CMR research.
- RF magnetic field gradient coils used to encode the position, thickness and orientation of the imaged slice
- Central computer to control the formation of images and the analysis of the MRI signal
- Console control to operate the MRI system: definition of sequences and geometries, data storage and handling
- Software programs for cardiac applications
- Contrast power injector
- Non-invasive blood pressure monitor (to be applied in pharmacological stress studies)
- Ideally, an MR compatible resuscitation system

1.5.2 Medical personnel

- Radiology technician/nurse
- Radiologist or cardiologist, ideally both working together as a team, in charge of study strategy design and image evaluation

1.5.3 Patient preparation

CMR is a prolonged examination (20 to 60 minutes) that requires patient cooperation. Claustrophobia, which occurs in a small percentage of cases, can lead to the cancellation of the study. Patients should be informed that they will have to remain motionless during the exam and that the system generates some loud noise. Young children or nervous patients should be sedated or given anaesthesia by an anaesthesiologist. The patient should avoid excessive swallowing, and respiration should be as regular as possible, avoiding large diaphragm movements (sighs, cough, etc.).

1.5.3.1 ECG synchronization

The most appropriate gating signal is the ECG R wave, since it permits to determine accurately the relation between MR images and the cardiac cycle. Surface ECG signal is obtained by means of electrodes placed on the skin which detect the electric activity of the heart. When the patient is placed inside the machine, where there is a very powerful magnetic field, respiratory movements and abrupt changes of magnetic gradient that occur during exam cause the generation of potentials induced between the electrodes. They are superimposed on the base ECG tracing, creating artifacts which can cause the signal to be unrecognizable. In addition, another artifact, especially if the system is 1.5 Tesla or higher, may be added, a phenomenon known as the magneto-hydrodynamic effect. When the blood cell particles with an electric charge (ions) move in a direction perpendicular to the magnetic field, they create additional electric potentials in the cardiovascular area resulting in the formation of a prolonged electric pulse which usually superimposes itself on the ECG T wave. Occasionally the intensity of the artifact is such that it creates a signal of the same amplitude as the R wave, causing problems to the algorithm detecting the synchronisation signal.

Artefacts superimposed on the ECG signal can become a significant practical problem, sometimes difficult to solve, but they can be minimized by taking into consideration some rules:

– Electrodes should be placed on those areas of the body that are the most likely to remain motionless, taking special care to avoid respiratory motion.

- Excessive distance between electrodes should be avoided.
- Care should be taken so that the potentials induced among the electrodes are parallel to the magnetic field lines of the machine in order to minimize its amplitude.
- Stretch out the electrode wires to the maximum.

In order to avoid the risk of the electrodes absorbing energy and heating up, which could damage the skin, electrodes that have been specially designed for use in MR systems should be used. In order to avoid eyes injure, which are especially sensitive to excessive radiofrequency irradiation, electrodes and their wires should not be placed near the head.

If obtaining of a proper register of the ECG signal becomes problematic, the pulse wave (oxymeter) signal amplitude can be used as a synchronizing tool. Nevertheless, it should be kept in mind that the temporary definition of the pulse wave is not as precise as the ECG R wave. To detect the pulse wave amplitude, capillary optic sensors are generally employed, and they should be placed on the fingertips, as long as they are well perfused.

1.5.3.2 Artefacts

Ferromagnetic material and paramagnetic substances generate severe image artefacts, known as magnetic susceptibility artefacts, due to local changes in the magnetic field around them, which are most pronounced in the images obtained by gradient-echo sequences. In

operated cardiac patients suture wire of the sternum (Figure 1.19.A) or valvular prostheses (Figure 1.19.B) are a frequent cause of artefacts. However, these artefacts are in most cases restricted to the region around the object. Thus, the evaluation of the rest of the image is usually not hampered.

1.5.3.3 Safety considerations

CMR is an examination technique that does not produce lesions in biological tissue. Contraindications for the study arise from the effect of the magnetic field on magnetic or metallic prosthesis or implants (Table 1.3). Thus, in CMR it is important to be aware that patients with implanted pacemakers or defibrillators should not undergo the MR examination, since the powerful magnetic field can interfere with the electronic components and cause them to function abnormally which might result in serious heart rhythm disturbances. Likewise, in patients with thermodilution catheters the electromagnetic field can cause overheating due to induction currents generated by the metal content of the catheters, which can cause serious burns, especially at the cutaneous insertion area of the catheter.

However, metal clips used to identify aorto-coronary by-pass grafts, suture wire for the sternum and vascular-coronary endoprosthesis (stents) do not represent a contraindication for an MR study[22]. It is also not contraindicated to study patients with valvular mechanical prosthesis, except in the case of the old Starr-Edwards model (Pre-6000), which has a high ferromagnetic content. The small torsion force that may be produced in the prosthesis, due to

FIGURE 1.19

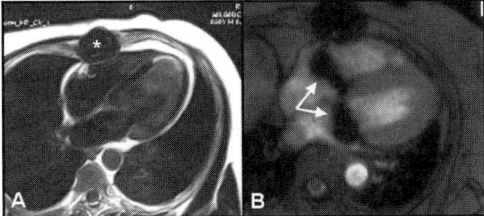

F. 1.19. A. Axial plane showing the artefact produced by the suture wire (asterisk). B. Axial plane in a patient with mitral and tricuspid metallic prostheses. See the artefact (arrows) produced by valvular prostheses, which is rather circumscribed, thus, allowing good quality images of the rest of structures.

Table 1.3 Contraindications for the practice of a magnetic resonance study

Pacemaker, implanted defibrillator or neurostimulator
Intracraneal iron clips
Metallic intraocular foreign body
Metallic fragment near a vital structure (projectile)
Cochlear implant or hearing aid
Starr-Edwards mitral valve prosthesis, model 6000 or earlier
Claustrophobia
Critical patient with a Swan-Ganz catheter
Pregnancy (relative: teratogenic effect not demonstrated)

the effect of the magnetic field, is much less than that which is generated by the mechanical force of the heartbeat. Concerning other new kinds of materials, the tendency of those to be implanted in the body is to avoid ferromagnetic material in order to prevent risks during MR examinations. However, it is advisable to consult up-to-date revisions of the listings of prostheses and implants published periodically in specialized journals in case an MR examination might be contraindicated[23].

1.6 Normal CMR anatomy

There are common pulse sequences for cardiovascular imaging, regardless of the MR system used, as well as anatomical image study planes that one should become familiar with. CMR allows the acquisition of slice planes in any orientation. However, it is advisable to perform the study in a standard way which facilitates appropriate image analysis.

A set of localising scout images in the three orthogonal planes (axial, sagittal, and coronal) is initially obtained (Figure 1.20). New planes can be prescribed from the scout images in order to obtained oblique planes orientated to the true cardiac axis. However, it has to be noted that excessive reliance on oblique planes or double obliquities may create serious difficulties with the interpretation of the relations of anatomic structures. Therefore, the more complicated the anatomic structure to be studied is (e.g., a complex congenital heart disease), the more necessary it is to undertake the study methodically, including standard orthogonal planes that are easily interpreted, in order to avoid confusion upon analysing anatomical relations.

1.6.1 Orthogonal planes

Mainly used to analyse anatomical relations of cardiovascular structures in morphological studies.

- Transverse or axial plane (Figures 1.21–1.28)
  It is especially useful to study the anatomic relations of cardiovascular structures by analysing images at consecutive levels.
- Sagittal plane (Figures 1.29–1.33)
  The sagittal plane allows the analysis of the right infundibulum and the main pulmonary artery in longitudinal views. It also permits a suitable study of the atrial septum, both cava veins and the thoracic descending aorta.
- Coronal plane (Figures 1.34–1.37)
  It allows the analysis of the relation of the trachea and the main bronchi to the cardiovascular structures. The left ventricular outflow tract and the vascular structures can be adequately seen.

1.6.2 Oblique planes

Oblique and double oblique planes orientated along the cardiac long/short axis are routinely used in CMR studies. Imperative in left ventricular (LV) function assessment, as well as in ischemic heart disease patients to perform perfusion and viability studies.

- Sagittal oblique planes
  A view displaying the whole thoracic aorta is obtained by a plane programmed on an

---

F. 1.20. Localising scout images in the 3 orthogonal planes. These are really fast acquisition images but with low spatial resolution. However, they are only used to prescribed the rest of the study.
AX, axial; COR, coronal; SAG, sagittal

F. 1.21. A coronal localizing image is used as anatomical reference for prescribing an axial SE sequence.

F. 1.22. Axial plane at the level of the supra-aortic arterial vessels.
CBA, common brachiocephalic artery; E, esophagous; LCA, left carotid artery; LSA, left subclavian artery; Tr, trachea;

F. 1.23. Axial plane at the level of the aortic arch.
AAch, aortic arch; IV, innominate vein; SVC, superior vena cava; Tr, trachea

F. 1.24. Axial at the level of great vessels.
AA, ascending aorta; DA, descending aorta; LB, left bronchus; LPA, left pulmonary artery; MPA, main pulmonary artery; RB, right bronchus; RPA, right pulmonary artery; SVC, superior vena cava

F. 1.25. Axial plane at the level of the left atrium.
AA, ascending aorta; AzV, azygous vein; DA, descending aorta; LA, left atrium; MPA, main pulmonary artery; RLPV, right lower pulmonary vein; SVC, superior vena cava

FIGURE 1.20

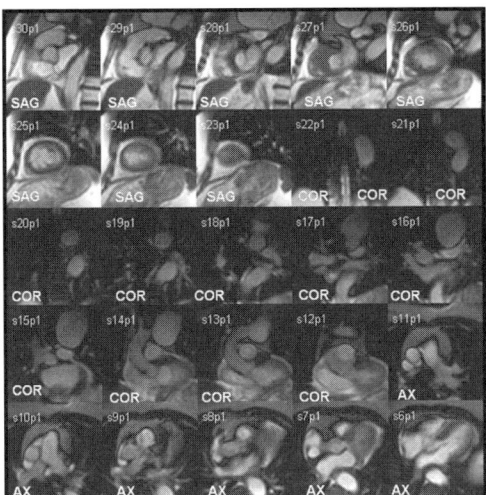

FIGURE 1.23

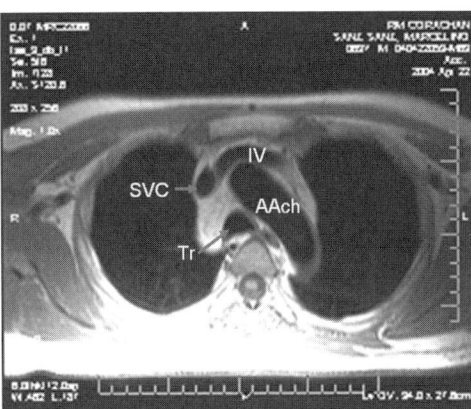

FIGURE 1.21

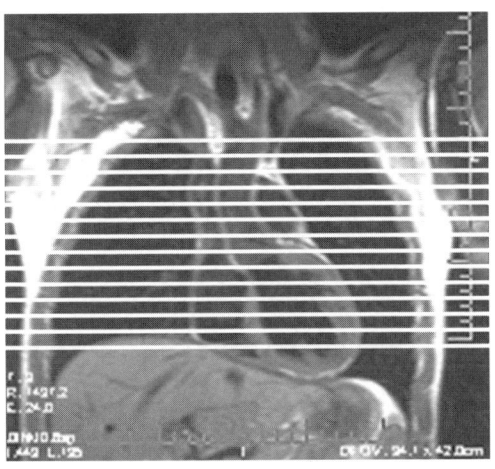

FIGURE 1.24

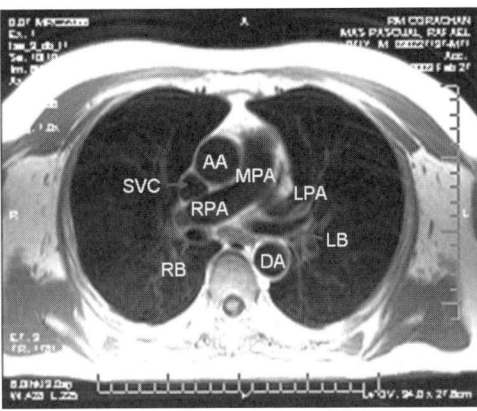

FIGURE 1.22

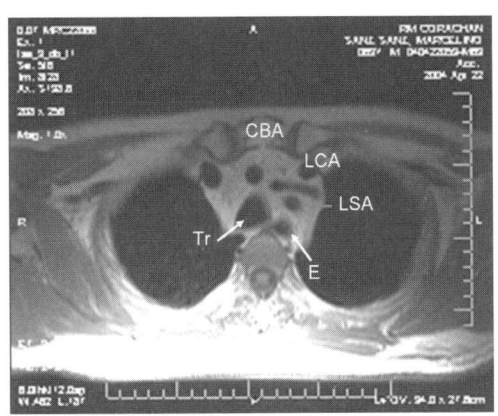

FIGURE 1.25

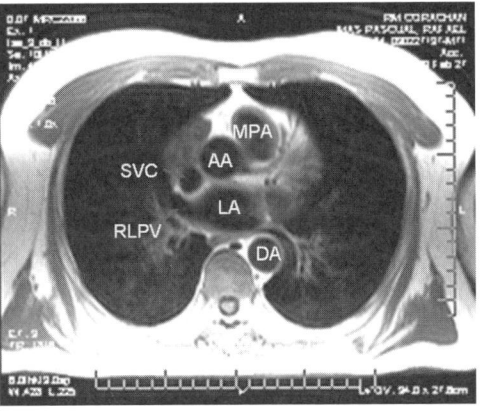

FIGURE 1.26

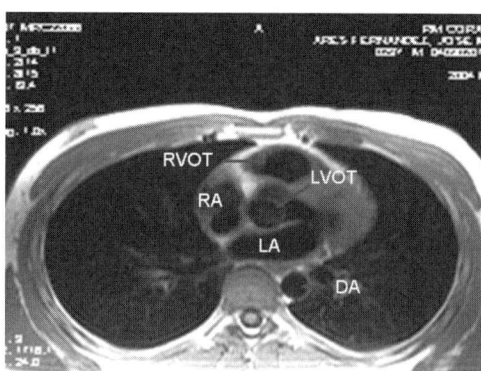

FIGURE 1.29

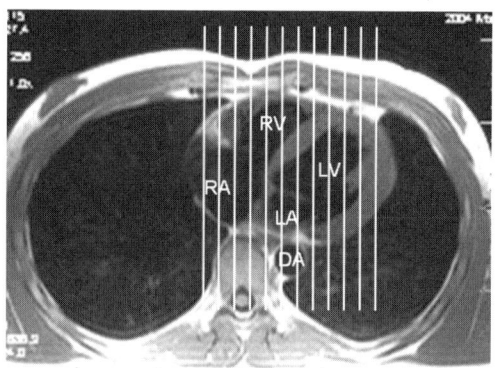

FIGURE 1.27

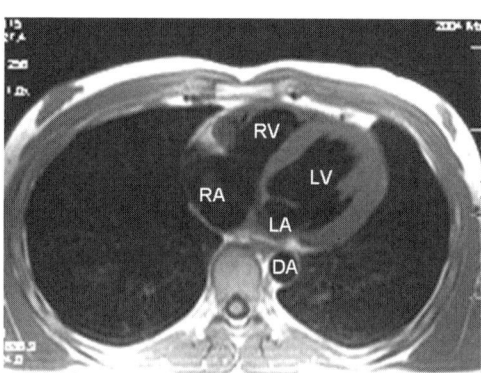

FIGURE 1.30

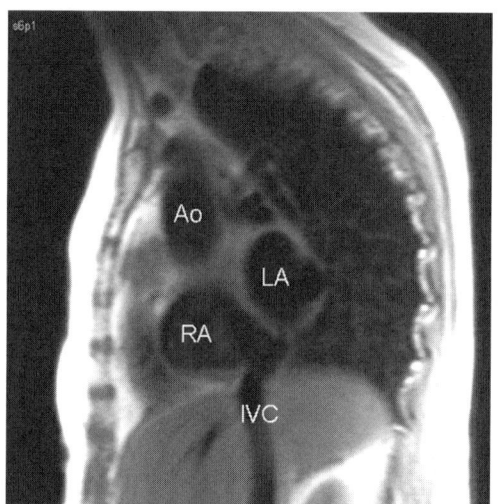

FIGURE 1.28

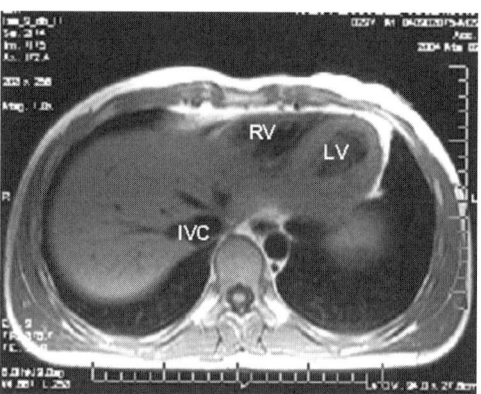

F. 1.26. Axial plane at the level of the ventricular outflow chambers.
DA, descending aorta; LA, left atrium; RA, right atrium; LVOT, left ventricle outflow tract; RVOT, right ventricle outflow tract

F. 1.27. Axial plane at the ventricular level.
DA, descending aorta; LA, left atrium; LV, left ventricle; RA, right atrium; RV, right ventricle

F. 1.28. Axial plane at the level of inferior vena cava.
IVC, inferior vena cava; LV, left ventricle; RV, right ventricle

F. 1.29. Axial localizing plane serve as a reference image for prescribing a sagittal SE sequence.

F. 1.30. Sagittal plane at the atrial level.
Ao, ascending aorta; IVC, inferior vena cava; LA, left atrium; RA, right atrium

FIGURE 1.31

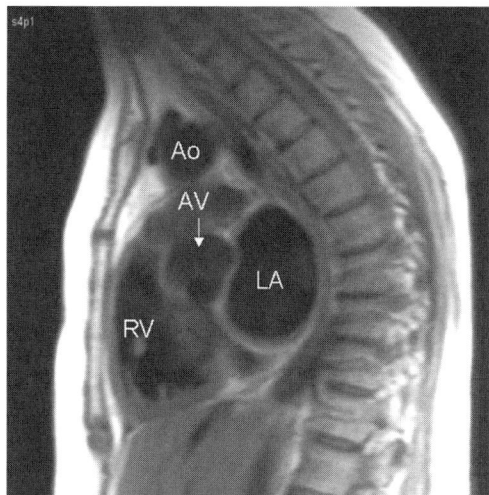

FIGURE 1.33

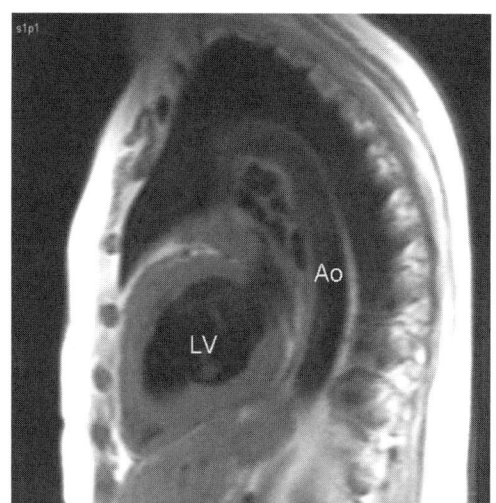

FIGURE 1.32

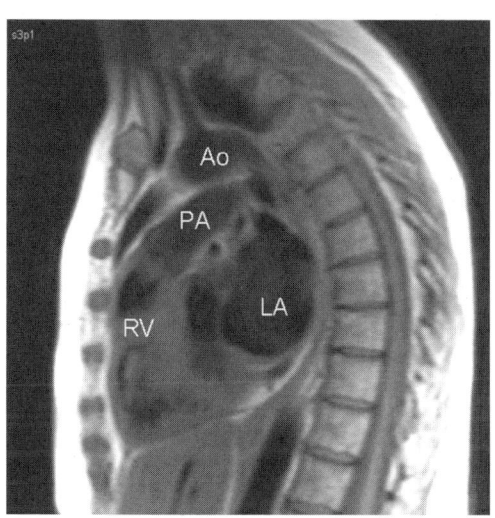

FIGURE 1.34

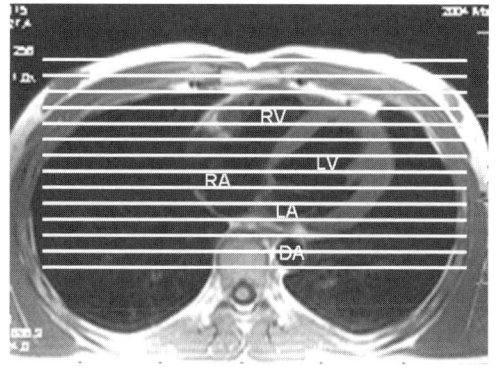

FIGURE 1.35

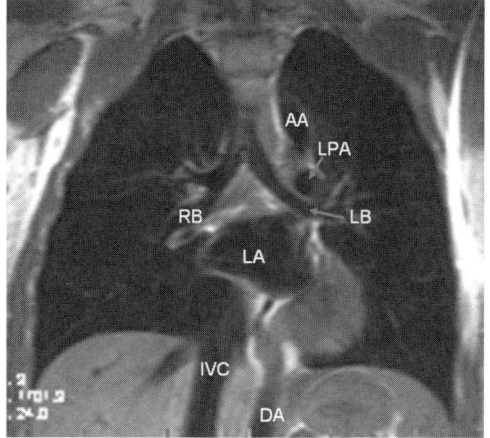

F. 1.31. Sagittal plane at the level of the aortic valve (AV).
Ao, aortic arch; LA, left atrium; RV, right ventricle

F. 1.32. Sagittal plane at the level of the right ventricular outflow tract.
Ao, aortic arch; LA, left atrium; PA, main pulmonary artery; RV, right ventricle

F. 1.33. Sagittal at the level of the left ventricle (LV).
Ao, descending aorta

F. 1.34. Axial localizing plane serve as a reference image for prescribing a coronal SE sequence.

F. 1.35. Coronal plane at the tracheal level.
IVC, inferior vena cava; DA, descending aorta; LB, left bronchus; LPA, left pulmonary artery; RB, right bronchus; AA, ascending aorta; LA, left atrium

FIGURE 1.36

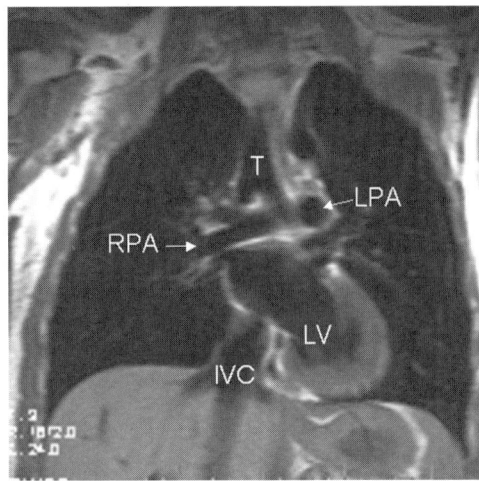

FIGURE 1.37

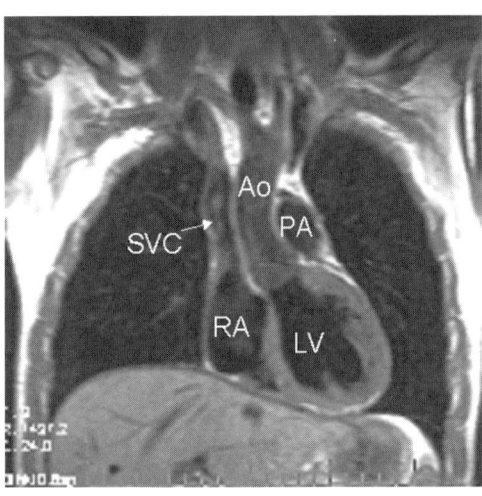

FIGURE 1.38

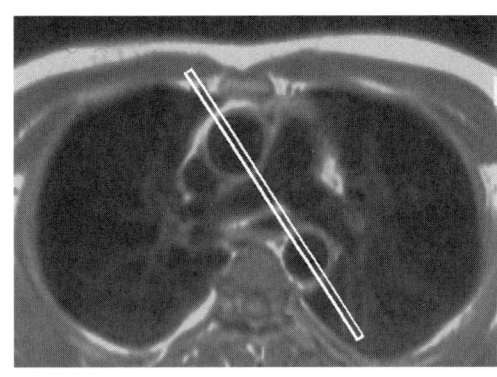

FIGURE 1.39

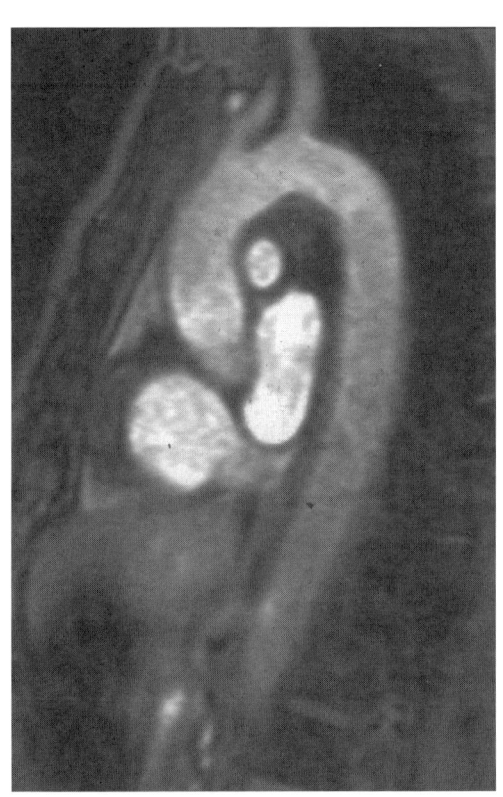

F. 1.36. Coronal plane at the level of the bifurcation of the pulmonary artery.
IVC, inferior vena cava; LPA, left pulmonary artery; LV, left ventricle; RPA, right pulmonary artery; T, trachea

F. 1.37. Coronal plane at the level of the left ventricular outflow tract.
Ao, ascending aorta; LV, left ventricle; PA, main pulmonary artery; RA, right atrium; SVC, superior vena cava

F. 1.38. Prescription of an oblique sagittal plane including the ascending and descending portions of the aorta.

F. 1.39. Oblique sagittal plane of the aorta on GRE obtained with the orientation described in the previous figure.

axial slice encompassing the planes of the ascending and descending portions of the aorta (Figures 1.38 and 1.39).

- Two-chamber plane

  From an axial scout showing right ventricle, left ventricle, and mitral valve (pseudo-four chamber), a two-chamber (2Ch) view of the left ventricle (vertical longitudinal) is obtained by prescribing a plane from the base, through the mitral valve, to the apex (Figure 1.40).

- Four-chamber plane: double oblique plane

  From the vertical longitudinal view (2Ch) a short-axis mid-ventricular plane (at the level of the papillary muscles) is obtained (Figure 1.41). Using both the 2Ch view and the mid short axis plane, an horizontal longitudinal view or four chamber plane (4Ch) is obtained, by transecting the mitral valve and the apex (Figure 1.42)

- Left ventricular "true" short axis: double oblique plane.

  A plane orthogonal to the longitudinal axis of the left ventricle, using both 2- and 4 Ch views (Figure 1.43).

FIGURE 1.42

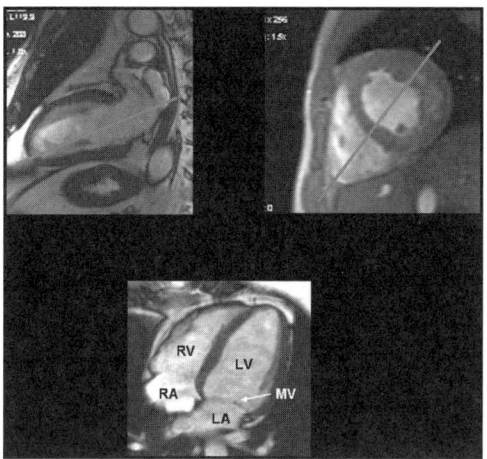

FIGURE 1.40

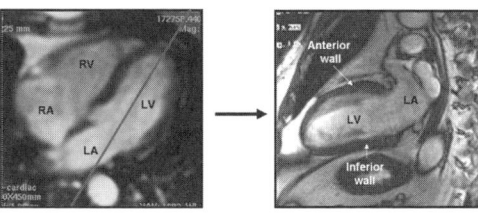

FIGURE 1.41

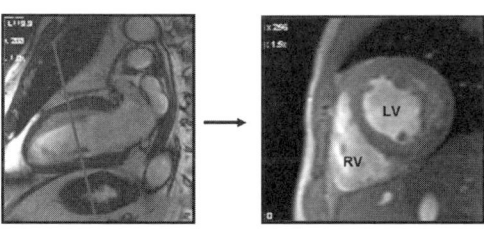

FIGURE 1.43

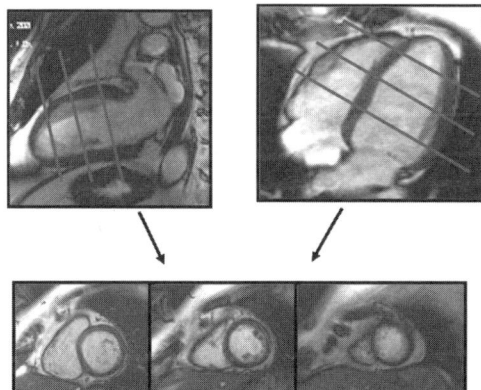

F. 1.40. On the left panel an axial plane serves as a localizer for prescribing an oblique plane oriented along the longitudinal axis of the left ventricle, in which the location of the apex and the base of the LV are taken as references. On the right the resulting vertical LV long-axis view.
LA, left atrium; LV, left ventricle; RA, right atrium; RV, right ventricle;

F. 1.41. Vertical long-axis image (on the left) is used to prescribe a short-axis plane at the mid-ventricular level (on the right).
LV, left ventricle; RV, right ventricle

F. 1.42. Using both short- (top right) and vertical long-axis (top left) images, an oblique slice oriented along the LV long-axis plane is prescribed. "True" LV horizontal long-axis plane (4 chamber) is obtained (bottom).
LA, left atrium; LV, left ventricle; MV, mitral valve; RA, right atrium; RV, right ventricle

F. 1.43. Double oblique plane oriented along LV short-axis is prescribed using both long-axis images, vertical (2 chamber view) (upper left) and horizontal (upper right). Bottom images showing short-axis images at 3 different levels.

FIGURE 1.44

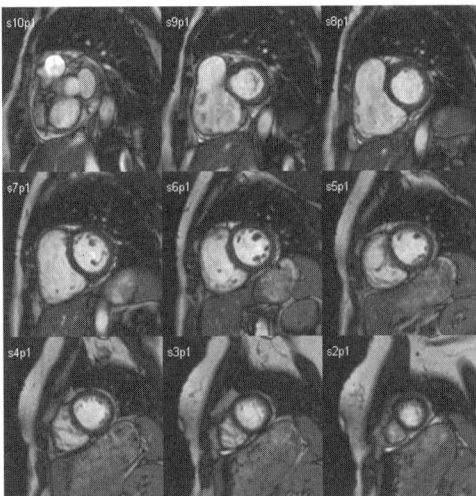

F. 1.44. A full set of short-axis images from the LV base to the apex covering the whole ventricular volumes.

A multislice study from the base to the apex covering the entire ventricles can then be prescribed in order to obtain the whole ventricular volumes (Figure 1.44).

References

1. Purcell EM, Torrey HC, Pound RV. Resonance absorption by nuclear magnetic moments in a solid. Physical Review 1946; 69:37.

2. Lauterbur PC. Image formation by induced local interactions: examples employing nuclear magnetic resonance. Nature 1973; 242:190–191.

3. Herfkens RJ, Higgins CB, Hricak H, et al. Nuclear magnetic resonance imaging of the cardiovascular system: normal and pathologic findings. Radiology 1983; 147:749–759.

4. Higgins CB, Caputo GR. Role of MR imaging in acquired and congenital cardiovascular disease. AJR Am J Roentgenol 1993; 161:13–22.

5. Pons Llado G, Carreras F, Guma JR, et al. [Uses of magnetic resonance in cardiology: initial experience in 100 cases]. Rev Esp Cardiol 1994; 47 Suppl 4:156–165.

6. The clinical role of magnetic resonance in cardiovascular disease. Task force of the European Society of Cardiology, in collaboration with the association of European Paediatric Cardiologists. European Heart Journal 1998; 19:19–39.

7. Pohost GM, Hung L, Doyle M. Clinical use of cardiovascular magnetic resonance. Circulation 2003; 108:647–653.

8. Sechtem U, Pflugfelder PW, White RD, et al. Cine MR imaging: potential for the evaluation of cardiovascular function. AJR Am J Roentgenol 1987; 148:239–246.

9. Pettigrew RI. Cardiovascular imaging techniques. In: Stark DD, Bradley WB, eds. Magnetic resonance imaging. St Louis: Mosby-year boook, 1992; 1605–1651.

10. Rebergen SA, van der Wall EE, Doornbos J, de Roos A. Magnetic resonance measurement of velocity and flow: technique, validation, and cardiovascular applications. Am Heart J 1993; 126:1439–1456.

11. Lotz J, Meier C, Leppert A, Galanski M. Cardiovascular flow measurement with phase-contrast MR imaging: basic facts and implementation. Radiographics 2002; 22:651–671.

12. Wilman AH, Riederer SJ, King BF, Debbins JP, Rossman PJ, Ehman RL. Fluoroscopically triggered contrast-enhanced three-dimensional MR angiography with elliptical centric view order: application to the renal arteries. Radiology 1997; 205:137–146.

13. Vignaux OB, Augui J, Coste J, et al. Comparison of single-shot fast spin-echo and conventional spin-echo sequences for MR imaging of the heart: initial experience. Radiology 2001; 219:545–550.

14. Chien D, Edelman RR. Ultrafast imaging using gradient echoes. Magn Reson Q 1991; 7:31–56.

15. Atkinson DJ, Edelman RR. Cineangiography of the heart in a single breath hold with a segmented turboFLASH sequence. Radiology 1991; 178:357–360.

16. Barkhausen J, Ruehm SG, Goyen M, Buck T, Laub G, Debatin JF. MR evaluation of ventricular function: true fast imaging with steady- state precession versus fast low-angle shot cine MR imaging: feasibility study. Radiology 2001; 219:264–269.

17. Lee VS, Resnick D, Bundy JM, Simonetti OP, Lee P, Weinreb JC. Cardiac function: MR evaluation in one breath hold with real-time true fast imaging with steady-state precession. Radiology 2002; 222:835–842.

18. Weiger M, Pruessmann KP, Boesiger P. Cardiac real-time imaging using SENSE. SENSitivity Encoding scheme. Magn Reson Med 2000; 43:177–184.

19. Simonetti OP, Kim RJ, Fieno DS, et al. An improved MR imaging technique for the visualization of myocardial infarction. Radiology 2001; 218:215–223.

20. Fenchel M, Helber U, Simonetti OP, et al. Multislice first-pass myocardial perfusion imaging: Comparison of saturation recovery (SR)-TrueFISP-two-dimensional (2D) and SR-TurboFLASH-2D pulse sequences. J Magn Reson Imaging 2004; 19:555–563.

21. Wetter DR, McKinnon GC, Debatin JF, von Schulthess GK. Cardiac echo-planar MR imaging: comparison of single- and multiple-shot techniques. Radiology 1995; 194:765–770.

22. Hug J, Nagel E, Bornstedt A, Schnackenburg B, Oswald H, Fleck E. Coronary arterial stents: safety and artifacts during MR imaging. Radiology 2000; 216:781–787.

23. Ahmed S, Shellock FG. Magnetic resonance imaging safety: implications for cardiovascular patients. J Cardiovasc Magn Reson 2001; 3:171–182.

24. Bottomley PA, Foster TH, Argersinger RE, Pfeifer LM. A review of normal tissue hydrogen NMR relaxation times and relaxation mechanisms from 1–100 MHz: dependence on tissue type, NMR frequency, temperature, species, excision, and age. Med Phys 1984; 11:425–448.

Ventricular Morphology and Function: Study of Cardiomyopathies

GUILLEM PONS-LLADÓ

2.1 Morphological Study of Heart Chambers

a. Left ventricle (LV)

The morphological assessment of the LV can be performed by either spin-echo (SE) T1-weighted ("black-blood") or gradient-echo (GRE) ("white-blood") sequences, both obtained during breath-hold. The first ones provide statical high-resolution images with excellent contrast between the myocardium and the intracavitary flow without the need for contrast agents[1] (Figure 2.1). The GRE sequences, used for the obtention of cine images, had shown a relatively low level of contrast, even when using fast imaging sequences (Figure 2.2). However, the introduction of new improved modalities of acquisition, as the segmented Steady-State Free Precession (SSFP) sequences, has greatly improved the image quality[2] (Figure 2.3), being the "white-blood" sequences widely used at present for the assessment of the LV, including the measurement of dimensions and wall thickness, and the calculation of functional parameters.

Whatever technique is used, and in order to get standardized and reproducible measurements, it is important to follow an acquisition strategy[3] allowing the obtention of slices on either longitudinal or transverse true anatomical planes of the LV. Since the long ventricular axis is not generally aligned within any of the natural planes of the body (Figure 2.4), it will be necessary to perform a series of angulations, the whole process including optimally 5 steps: (1) first, one of the scout axial planes is selected where an estimate of the position of the base and the apex of the LV can be taken (Figure 2.5); by using these two reference points (line on Figure 2.5) we will prescribe on this plane a single slice, that will give (2) an oblique sagittal image oriented on a vertical longitudinal plane (VLP) of the LV (2-chamber view), including the anterior wall, the ventricular apex and the inferior wall (Figure 2.6); then, a natural complementary orientation would be an horizontal plane, orthogonal to the vertical one, but for an optimal orientation a previous intermediate step is recommended: it consists of (3) a transverse plane of the ventricles (Figure 2.7) taken on the VLP (vertical line on Figure 2.6); now, by using the two views described in steps 2 and 3, a plane is prescribed with a double angulation: orthogonal to the VLP (horizontal line on Figure 2.6), on one side, and then aligned with the maximal diameter of the right ventricle on the transverse plane (line on Figure 2.7), this giving (4) a true horizontal longitudinal plane (HLP) of the LV (4-chamber view of the heart), including the septal wall, the ventricular apex and the lateral free wall (Figure 2.8); a final step is the obtention of (5) multiple transverse planes of the ventricles (Figure 2.9) with an orientation parallel to the atrio-ventricular plane (lines on Figure 2.8).

The obtention of this series of sequences can be performed at present, by using, for instance, SSFP cine sequences with breath-hold acquisition, in less than 10 minutes. A strict routine following this protocol is highly recommended as a part of most CMR studies, as it provides a complete dataset containing accurate and reliable information on the LV, both morfological and functional.

Basic measurements of the LV can be performed on these standard anatomically-oriented views, as the maximal transverse dimension of the LV, with a mean normal value in adult men of 50 mm (upper 95% limit: 59 mm); and, in adult women, 46 mm (upper 95% limit: 51 mm); or the diastolic septal and wall thickness, with normal means of 10 mm (upper 95% limit: 12 mm) in men, and 9 mm (upper 95% limit: 10 mm) in women[4]. Moreover, in a good deal of heart diseases, a complete morphological study of the LV must include a determination of the left ventricular mass (LVM). It can be obtained by means of an appropriate software allowing the computation of the diastolic endocardial and epicardial contours of the ventricle (Figure 2.10) on the series of transverse planes covering the whole extension of the chamber, from base to apex. A standard planning of the sequences, with slice thickness between 8–10 mm, interslice gap of up to 5 mm and in-plane resolution (pixel size) up to 3 mm, allow a reliable calculation of LVM in practice[5]. The method has shown a high degree of accuracy in animal experimental studies[6] and is considered at present as a reference against which other methods can be compared: when echocardiography, the most widely-used technique for the estimation of LVM in practice, has been tested, a significant variation in LVM estimates

from the direct measurement of CMR has been observed[7,8], which is not surprising, provided the diverse geometric assumptions involved in the calculation by ultrasound. The excellent reproducibility of LVM measurement by MRI should be noted, which has important practical applications in those cases in which a series of determinations of this parameter are required, particularly when the objective is to estimate evolutionary changes of ventricular hypertrophy[9]. Values for LVM estimated by CMR on normal populations have been published[3,4,10–12], that can be used as a reference to detect abnormal left ventricular hypertrophy in practice (Table 2.1).

b. Right ventricle (RV)

Due to the complex morphology of the RV, it is necessary to consider in its evaluation two anatomical regions: the inflow and outflow chambers. In axial slices the limit between both is determined by the change in configuration of the chamber, from triangular at the inflow chamber (Figure 2.1) to circular shaped in the outflow chamber (Figure 2.11), situated above. The outflow portion of the ventricle is also easily imaged in its longitudinal plane by means of sagittal views (Figure 2.12). Based on these images it is possible to determine the righ ventricular wall thickness, which in normal individuals is 3 mm (upper 95% limit: 5 mm) in diastolic images, as well as the maximum diameters of the chamber, the normal values being 32 mm (upper 95% limit: 42 mm) in the inflow chamber, and 26 mm (upper 95% limit: 34 mm) in the outflow portion[13].

It is also possible to determine the right ventricular mass (RVM) by applying the method of summation of transverse planes in a similar way to the calculation of LVM (Figure 2.10), and on the same set of images, tracing in this case the endocardial and epicardial contours of the RV (Figure 2.13). The method has been shown highly accurate in animal experimental studies[14]. Normal values of RVM have been published[3,11], absolute mean values ranging between 50 g (upper 95% limit: 70 g) for adult men to 40 g (upper 95% limit: 55 g) for women. As expected due to the particularly complex morphology of the right ventricular cavity, this method is less reproducible than in the case of the LVM[15], which may have consequences on sample size of

FIGURE 2.1

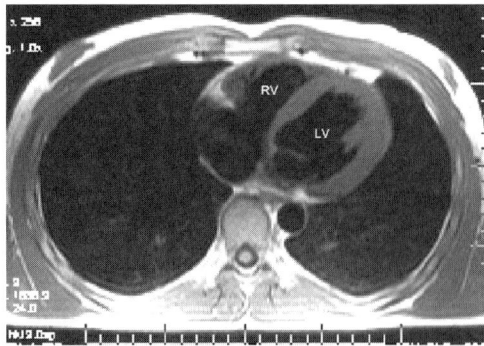

FIGURE 2.4

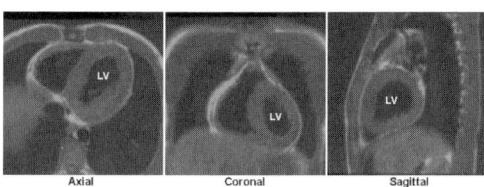

FIGURE 2.2

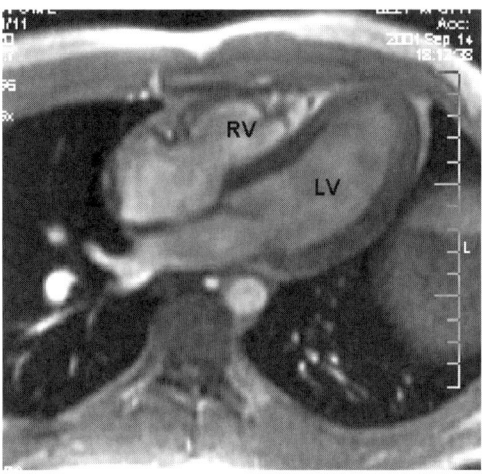

FIGURE 2.5

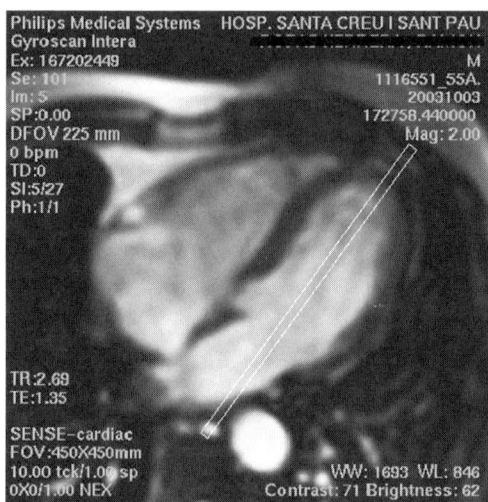

FIGURE 2.3

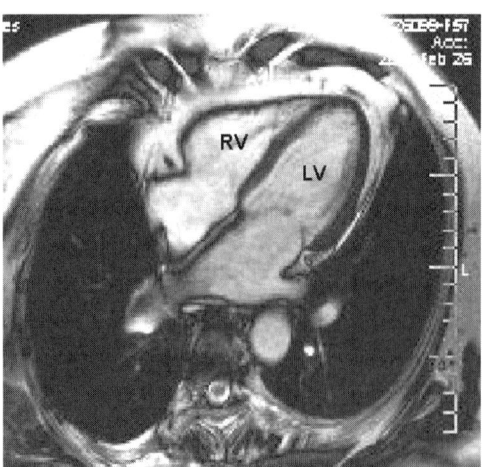

F. 2.1. Axial SE T1w image at the level of the right (RV) and left ventricle (LV). Note the virtual absence of signal of the blood, the intermediate signal intensity of the myocardial walls, and the high intensity corresponding to the adipose tissue.

F. 2.2. Axial GRE image from a series of Fast-Cine. Note the high signal intensity of blood in these sequences.

F. 2.3. Axial image from a Steady-State Free Precession (SSFP) sequence. Note the increase in contrast between structures, particularly blood and myocardium, with respect to conventional GRE sequences.

F. 2.4. SE T1w images on pure axial, coronal and sagittal planes, every one of them including the left ventricle (LV) in non-standard views.

F. 2.5. Axial scout plane where a longitudinal view of the LV is prescribed encompassing the apex and the mid point of the base of the ventricle.

FIGURE 2.6

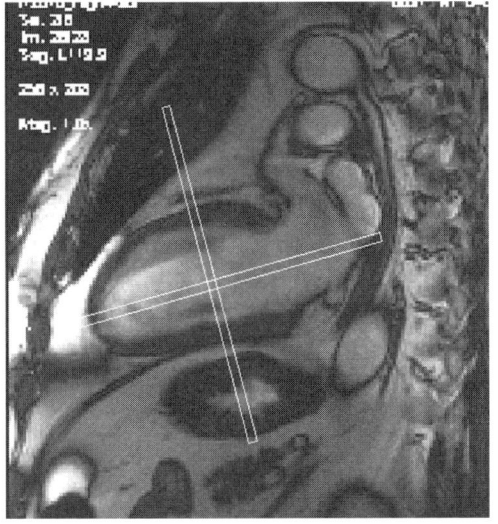

FIGURE 2.7

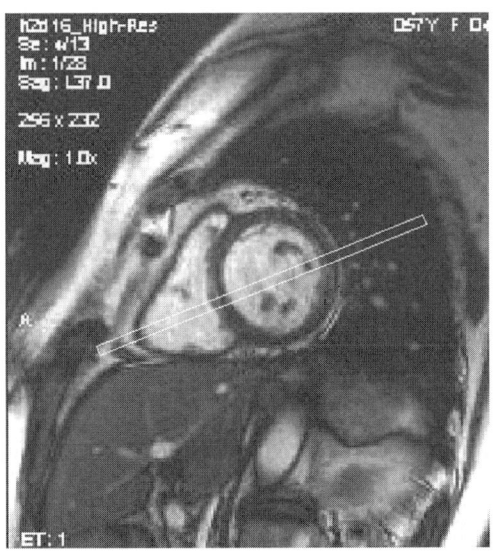

FIGURE 2.8

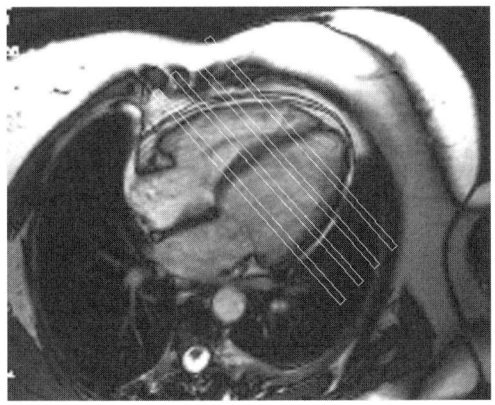

FIGURE 2.9

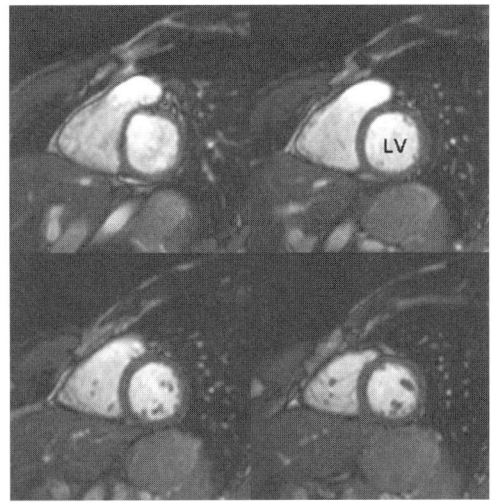

FIGURE 2.10

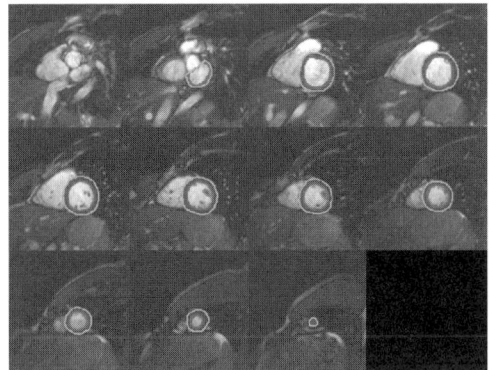

F. 2.6.   Vertical longitudinal plane of the LV (2-chamber view).

F. 2.7.   Transverse plane of the LV (Short-axis view).

F. 2.8.   Horizontal longitudinal plane of the LV (4-chamber view).

F. 2.9.   Series of parallel short-axis views of the LV.

F. 2.10. A complete series of short-axis views of the LV, from base to apex, where the endo- and epicardial contours have been manually traced in those images including these structures.

Table 2.1 Normal values of LVM (in g) as estimated by CMR: mean (upper 95% limit) absolute and indexed (by body surface area) values.

	Men		Women	
	Absolute	Indexed	Absolute	Indexed
Lorenz et al[3]	178 (238)	91 (113)	125 (175)	79 (95)
Marcus et al[10]	142 (182)	71 (88)	102 (134)	58 (79)
Sandstede et al[11]	155 (191)	78 (96)	110 (142)	65 (81)
Salton et al[4]	155 (201)	78 (95)	103 (134)	61 (75)
Alfakih et al[12]	133 (181)	65 (83)	90 (114)	52 (67)

FIGURE 2.11

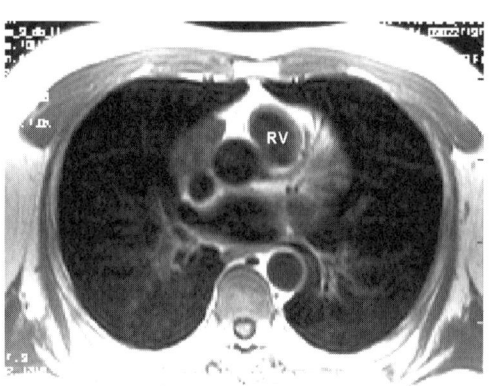

FIGURE 2.12

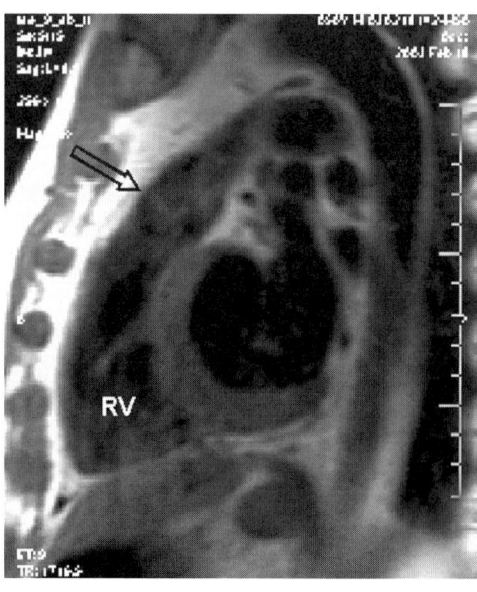

FIGURE 2.13

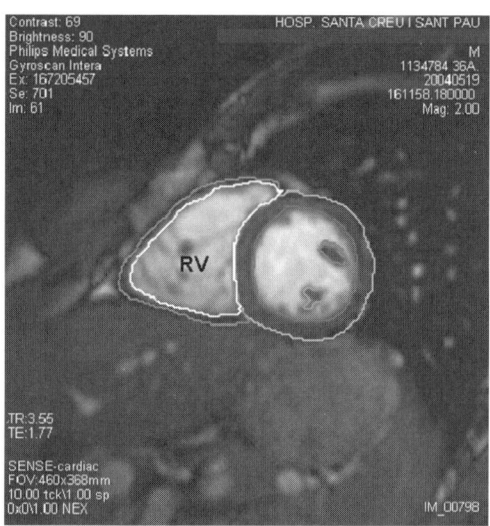

F. 2.11. Axial SE T1w plane at the level of the outflow tract on the right ventricle (RV).

F. 2.12. Sagittal SE T1w plane showing a longitudinal view of the outflow portion of the RV. The arrow points to the plane of the pulmonary valve.

F. 2.13. One of a series of short-axis planes where the endo- and epicardial contours of the RV have been traced, in addition to the ones of the LV.

populations in follow-up studies. This limitation is, however, less relevant in clinical practice, where the measurement of RVM is not routinely used.

2.2 Ventricular Function

a. Left ventricular function

MRI permits an accurate estimation of the volume of the left ventricular cavity by the acquisition of a series of parallel cine sequences, preferably SSFP with breath-hold[2], following the strategy described above (Figures 2.8–2.9) and selecting not only the end-diastolic (Figure 2.10), but also the end-systolic frames for tracing the endocardial contours (Figure 2.14). Once the end-diastolic and end-systolic volumes are obtained, then the left ventricular ejection fraction is easily derived. This study of ventricular volumes and function may be optimized by considering that, as with any process of image acquisition in CMR, a compromise exists that involves the total number of slices and the spatial and temporal resolution of the images, which, in the end, determines the number and duration of breath-hold periods from the patient. In order to simplify the process of acquisition, the number of transverse slices required to cover the whole extension of the LV may be reduced without penalty by increasing the interslice gap up to 15 mm[16], this allowing a reduction from 9–10 to 6–7 slices, in case of a non enlarged ventricular chamber. On the other hand, the reliability of the calculation of volumes and ejection fraction, is very sensitive to spatial and, particularly, to temporal resolution, a pixel size between 1 and 2 mm and temporal resolutions between 21 and 45 msec being recommended for an appropriate accuracy[4]. This means, in practice, to use matrix sizes not lower that 256 pixels, and number of phases per cardiac cycle of at least 16 (Cines 2.1 and 2.2 on CD). Finally, the process of calculation of volumes may be also simplified by not considering the papillary muscles and trabeculae that, in purity, should be subtracted from the total left ventricular volume (Figure 2.10). This reduces the time consumed in the analysis while not significantly altering the calculation of volumes and, particularly, ejection fraction[17].

The calculation of ventricular volumes and function is optimally performed by this method of summation of transverse slices of the left ventricle, and it is considered as a reference standard[4]. Several studies on normal individuals[3,4,11,12] have established that the mean normal value of left ventricular ejection fraction is 0.67 (lower 95% limit: 0.58). A fast evaluation of these parameters can be also obtained by simple plannimetry on longitudinal views of the LV, in a similar way to two-dimensional echocardiography (Figure 2.15). Although the method is still subject to the limitations of geometric assumptions, is an acceptable alternative to volumetric methods for the estimation of function[18] and even mass of the LV[7], at least in routine CMR exams where these data are not a main concern. Important to note is, however, that planar and volumetric methods cannot be considered interchangeable for a given patient[18].

Of particular interest in patients with ischemic heart disease is the assessment of regional left ventricular function. It can be easily estimated by visualization of short-axis cine sequences of the LV (Cine 2.3 on CD), where attention must be paid to basal wall thickness, systolic thickening and endocardial inward motion on every segment of the LV. A proposal for a unitary method of division (and nomenclature) in 17 segments of the LV has been made[19] that requires the analysis of 3 equidistant transverse short-axis planes and one longitudinal plane of the LV (Figure 2.16). Any degree of regional systolic dysfunction, either hypokinesia, akinesia, or dyskinesia, should be readily detected by a trained observer on this qualitative basis. There is, however, software equipment available to quantitatively estimate the extension and degree of regional myocardial disfunction by measurement of wall thickening (Figure 2.17). The tedious large amount of measurements on the digitized images that are required for these calculations when performed manually may be considerably alleviated by the application of semiautomated contour detection algorithms[20].

b. Right ventricular function

The set of cine sequences oriented on transverse short-axis planes of the ventricles (Figures 2.8 and 2.9) contains information from which to derive volume calculations of both the LV

FIGURE 2.14

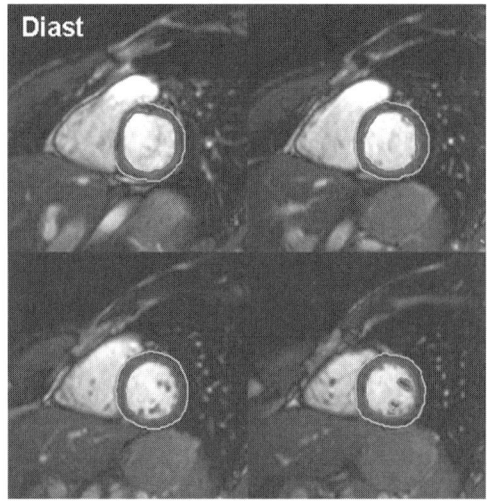
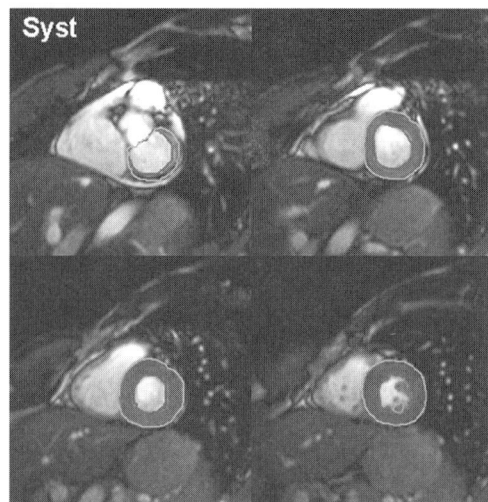

FIGURE 2.15

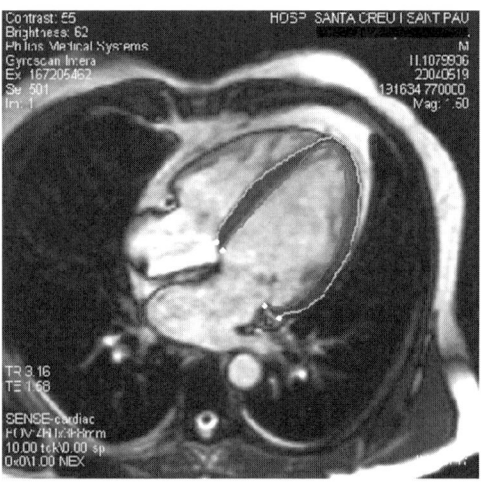
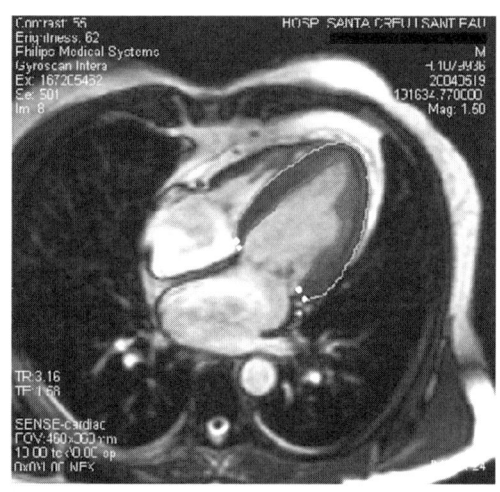

FIGURE 2.16

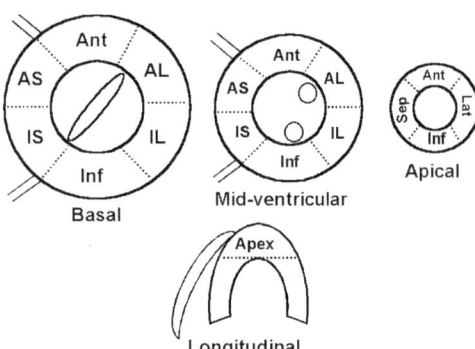

F. 2.14. Endo- and epicardial contours of the LV traced on a series of short-axis slices at both end-diastolic (left panel) and end-systolic (right) frames.

F. 2.15. Endo- and epicardial contours of the LV traced on a 4-chamber view both on end-diastolic (left panel) and end-systolic (right) frames.

F. 2.16. Model of 17-segment division of the LV.

F. 2.17. Computer-aided analysis of regional wall motion. An end-diastolic (upper left panel) and end-systolic (upper right) frames of a short-axis slice of the LV are shown where, after a tracing of the endo- and epicardial contours, a dedicated software (MASS, Medical Imaging Solutions, Leiden, The Netherlands) presents, by means of a radial analysis, a series of curves (lower panel) corresponding, in this case, to the time course over a cardiac cycle of wall thickness in every one of 6 segments at that particular short-axis plane. Note that there is reduced wall thickening at the anterior (solid arrow) and at the infero-septal (open arrow) segments, as seen on the corresponding curves below.

FIGURE 2.17

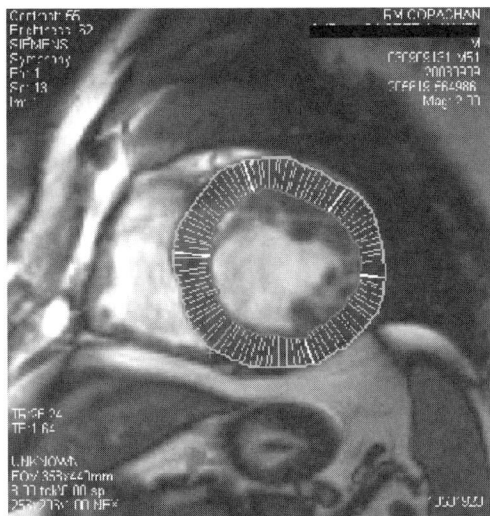 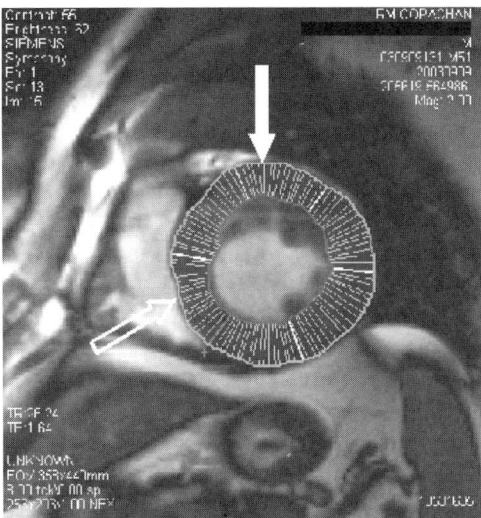

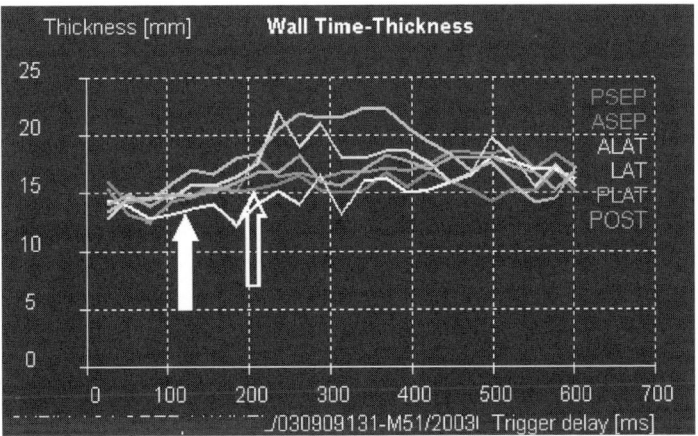

FIGURE 2.18

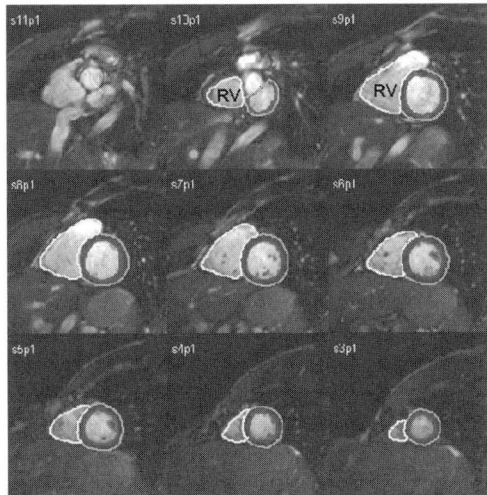 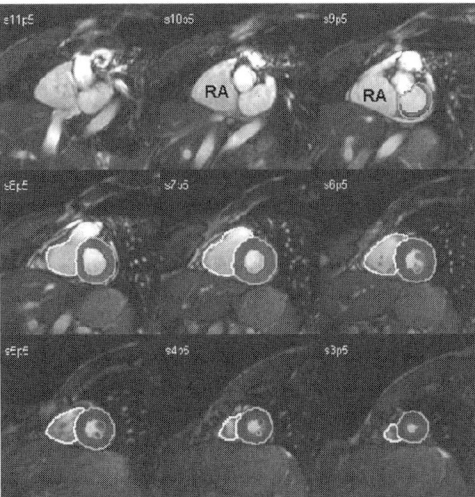

F. 2.18. End-diastolic (left panel) and end-systolic (right) frames from a complete series of short-axis views of the ventricles. In addition to the contours of the LV, the endocardial limits of the RV have also been traced. Care has been taken not to include as parts of the RV areas displaying in fact the right atrium (RA) (see text for details).

(Figure 2.14), and also the RV, by tracing, in this case, the appropriate end-diastolic and end-systolic endocardial contours (Figure 2.18). It is important to consider that, particularly in normally contracting hearts, a significant longitudinal displacement of the atrio-ventricular plane towards the apex may occur, which can cause the RV be imaged on end-diastole at the most basal planes (left panel on Figure 2.18), while these same slices at end-systole display the right atrial cavity (right panel on Figure 2.18). To pay close attention to this point is essential for an accurate measurement of volumes and function of the RV. It is useful, in this sense, to examine carefully the wall of the chamber, that is trabeculated in the case of the ventricle, and smooth when it corresponds to the atrium, or, also, to take into account that an apparent increase in the area of the RV from end-diastole to end-systole probably indicates that the right atrium is actually imaged in the systolic frame.

Calculation of volumes of the RV by this method has shown a good degree of accuracy with actual volumes determined on cadaveric human casts[21], reference values having been reported in clinical studies[3,11,12], where it has been established a normal mean value for right ventricular ejection fraction of 0.61 (lower 95% limit: 0.47). Nevertheless, volume calculations of the RV have shown a lower reproducibility than those obtained in the case of the LV[15], probably due to the difficulties arising from the delineation of the contours of the RV, as mentioned above. For this reason, alternative approaches have been tested, as is the tracing of the endocardial contours of the RV on strictly axial planes, rather than on short-axis slices, the former showing better inter- and intraobserver reproducibility in volume measurements[22].

In contrast with the LV, and provided the complex geometric shape of the RV, calculations of volume and function can not be reliably made on single longitudinal planes of the cavity.

2.3 Cardiomyopathies

a. Dilated cardiomyopathy (DCM)

The diagnosis of DCM is generally made by echocardiography that can realiably estimate the dimensions, volume and ejection fraction of the LV on most clinical instances. However, comparison studies between ultrasound and CMR[18] have shown that, at least with respect to conventional biplane echocardiographic methods, calculation of volumes and ejection fraction of the LV significantly differ from those estimated by volumetric CMR methods, this eventually leading to an incorrect classification of patients with DCM in terms of degree of severity of ventricular dysfunction. Thus, CMR has to be considered in diagnostic and, particularly, follow-up studies of these patients, where it has shown to perform efficiently[23]. Also, CMR has a definite role in research studies, since measurements of changes in these parameteres are more reproducible than with other techniques, and the required sample size is substantially smaller[24].

Patients with DCM usually present with signs and symptoms secondary to advanced left ventricular dysfunction, without a history suggestive of coronary artery disease (CAD). Despite of this, to rule out an ischemic origin of the myocardial damage is an important step of the diagnostic workup in a good deal of these patients, this usually requiring invasive coronary angiography. Since the demostration that scarring due to a previous myocardial necrosis may be reliably identified by contrast-enhanced CMR[25], interest arouse on the technique as a potential tool to distinguish dilated from ischemic cardiomyopathy. Early studies[26] reported that, using segmented inversion-recovery GRE sequences, patients with DCM showed complete absence of delayed myocardial contrast enhancement, while those with CAD presented with regional hyperenhancement indicating myocardial scarring (Figure 2.19). Studies on larger series of patients with DCM[27], however, have shown that nearly one third of cases present with some kind of contrast enhancement, appearing as patchy or midwall longitudinal striae (Figure 2.20), clearly different, in any case, from the extensive endocardial or transmural distribution seen in patients with CAD, and similar to the myocardial fibrosis found in autopsy studies of patients with DCM.

A particular type of cardiomyopathy is the so-called isolated left ventricular non compaction, a rare congenital defect of the endomyocardial morphogenesis with a poor prognosis[28].

FIGURE 2.19

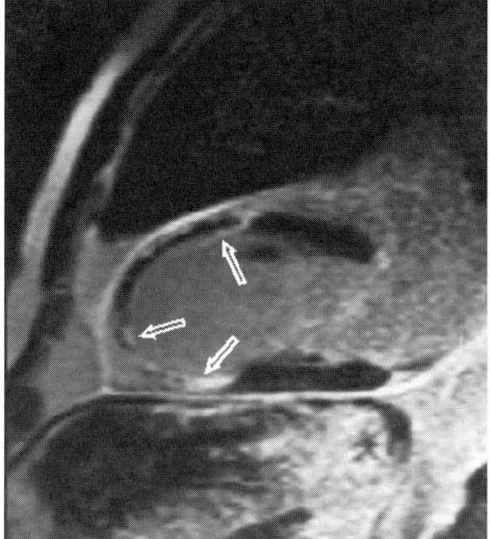
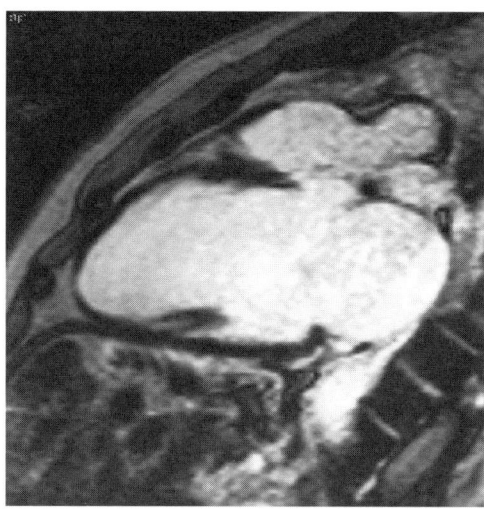

FIGURE 2.20

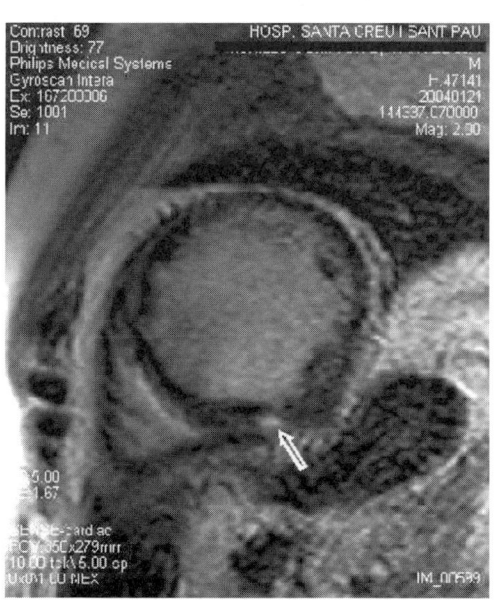
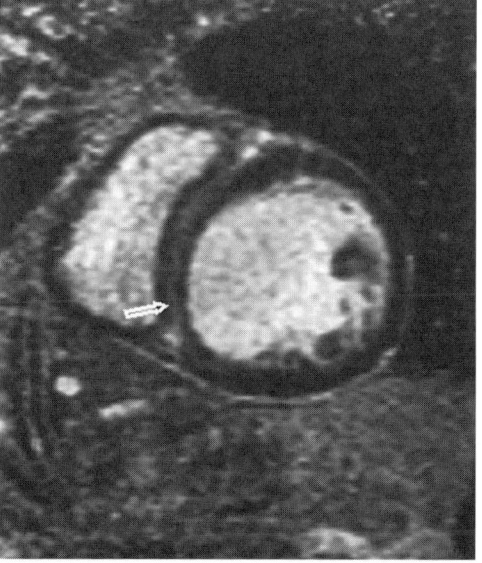

F. 2.19. Vertical long-axis views of the LV from a segmented inversion-recovery GRE sequence obtained late (15 min) after the administration of gadolinium. The left panel corresponds to a patient with ischemic heart disease, showing extensive myocardial scarring evidenced by delayed contrast enhancement (arrows). At right, an image from a patient with DCM, without myocardial contrast enhancement.

F. 2.20. Examples of delayed contrast enhancement found in DCM: arrows point to a focal (left) and to a longitudinal striated pattern of enhancement (right).

CMR is useful for the diagnosis as it clearly depicts the different features of the two layers in the left ventricular wall: the outer wall, thin and compacted, and the inner layer, spongy, densely trabeculated and noncompacted[29] (Figure 2.21 and Cine 2.4 on CD).

b. Hypertrophic cardiomyopathy (HCM)

The diagnostic role of echocardiography in this disease is not disputed as it permits not only to detect the presence and the extension of ventricular hypertrophy, but also to assess the

FIGURE 2.21

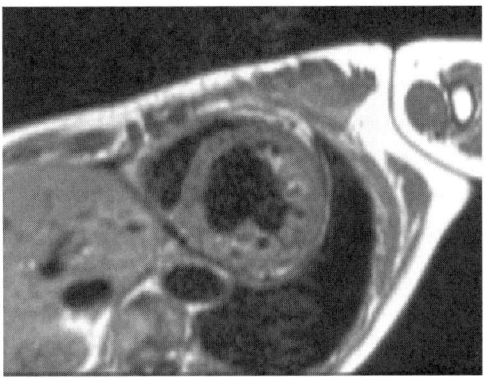

FIGURE 2.22

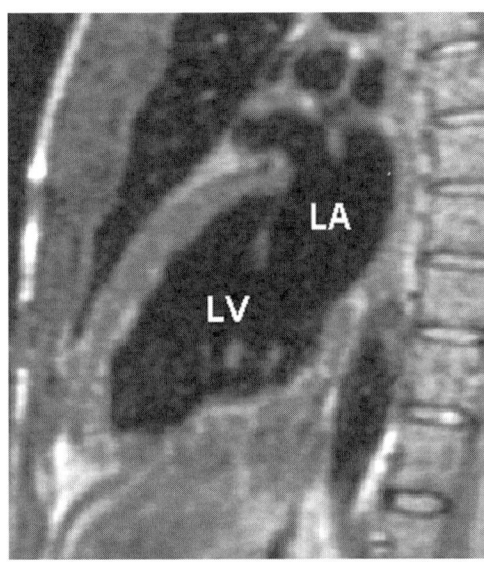
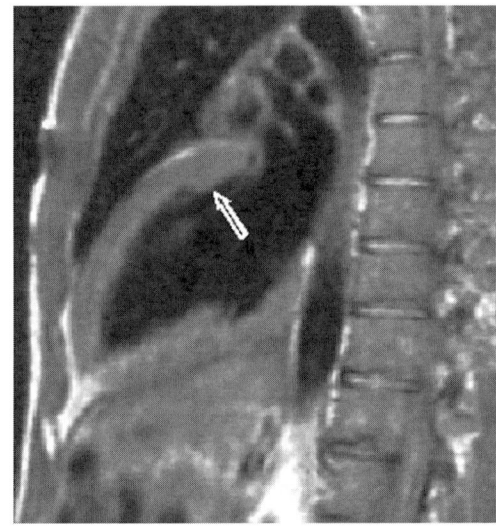

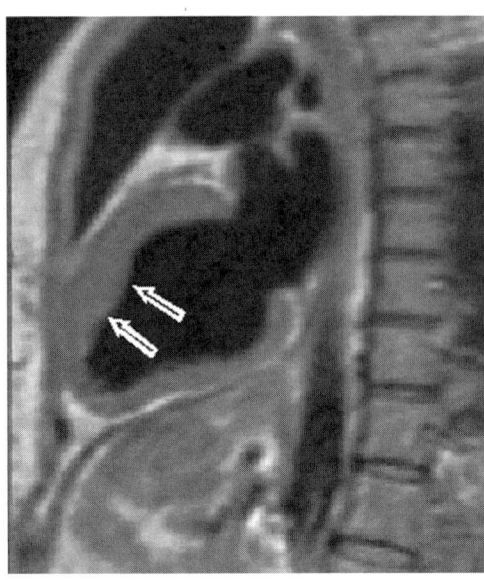
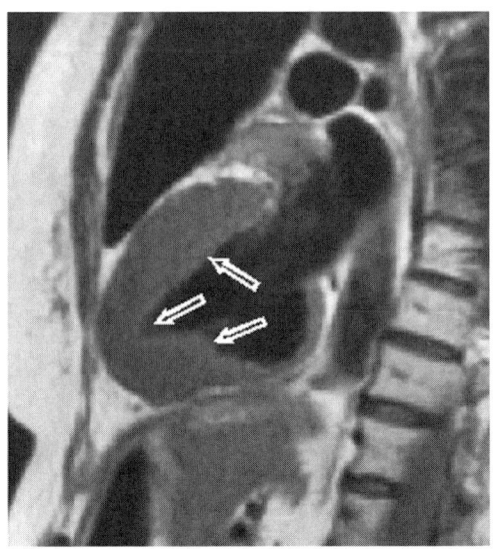

F. 2.21. Short-axis view on SE T1w in a case of left ventricular non compaction: observe the densely trabeculated component of the free wall of the LV.

F. 2.22. Examples from 4 different cases, all of them imaged with SE T1w sequences on vertical longitudinal views. Besides a normal subject (top left), different degrees of hypertrophy (arrows) are clearly depicted in patienmts with HCM, giving an accurate asessment of the extension of the disease in every case.

FIGURE 2.23

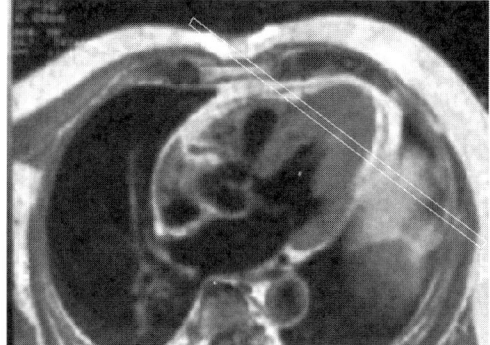

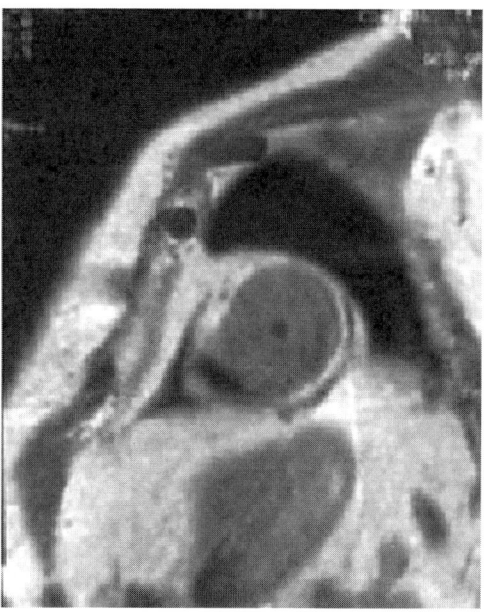

F. 2.23. Apical HCM: SE T1w sequences on axial (left panel) and short-axis (right) orientations, the latter obtained at the apical level of the LV (lines on the left panel).

degree of dynamic obstruction to flow, if present, and an eventual diastolic dysfunction of the LV. There are, however, known limitations of ultrasound in certain patients, due to inappropriate acoustic windows, that lead to the visualization of only part of all segments of the LV[30]. Provided that, in HCM, the process may be confined to specific regions of the LV which may be eventually not visualized by ultrasound, then CMR, with its ability to image the LV in all its planes without restriction (Figure 2.22 and Cine 2.5 on CD) becomes a valid alternative, particularly in some forms of the disease, as is the apical type (Figure 2.23) not rarely missed by echo-cardiography[31].

The dynamic functional components of HCM, as the outflow obstruction or the diastolic dysfunction, are not so reliably assessed by CMR, compared with Doppler-echocardiography. However, the presence of subaortic dynamic obstruction can be revealed by a signal void due to turbulent flow on longitudinal cine sequences including the left ventricular outflow tract (Cine 2.6 on CD).

Again, contrast techniques oriented to detect the presence of myocardial scar tissue have been useful when applied to patients with HCM. In contrast to DCM, here most patients (nearly 80%) present with some degree of late

enhancement, mainly implying the most hypertrophied segments[32], and thought to be due to myocardial fibrosis secondary to replacement scarring[33]. The extension and distribution of hyperenhancement is variable, although a fairly common finding is a pattern of distribution at the junctions of the inter-ventricular septum and the right ventricular free wall[32–34] (Figure 2.24). Importantly, the extent of hyperenhancement is associated with progressive forms of HCM and markers of sudden death[34].

Additionally, late contrast enhancement studies are helpful in those patients who have been submitted to alcohol septal ablation[35], where the area of subsequent myocardial necrosis is clearly delineated (Figure 2.25, and Cine 2.7 on CD).

c. Restrictive cardiomyopathy (RCM)

There are no distinctive morphological features of RCM at CMR studies, which also holds true for other diagnostic methods. This is particularly the case in idiopathic RCM, where there is no hypertrophy nor dilatation of the ventricles, but a profound primary diastolic dysfunction leading to indirect findings at CMR, as dilatation of both atria or pericardial effusion (Figure 2.26). Importantly, systolic

FIGURE 2.24

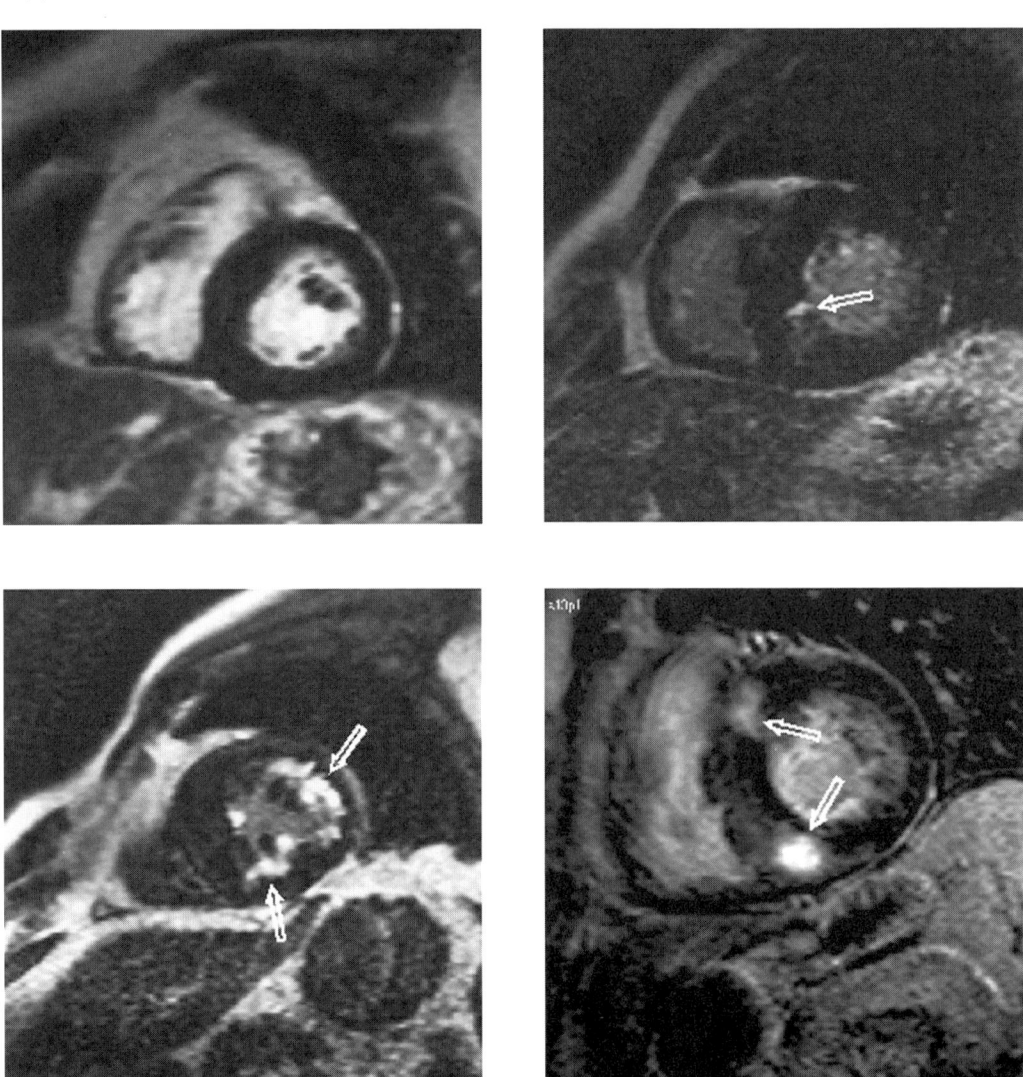

F. 2.24. Examples from 4 different patrients with HCM, in whom short-axis views of the LV have been obtained by means of a segmented inversion-recovery GRE sequence obtained late (15 min) after the administration of gadolinium. Different degrees of delayed contrast enhancement (arrows) can be observed, from none (top left), to unifocal (top right), confluent multifocal (bottom left), or located at the ventricular junctions (bottom right).

FIGURE 2.25

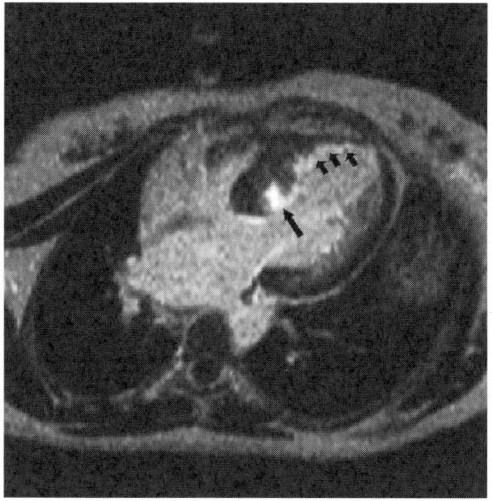

FIGURE 2.26

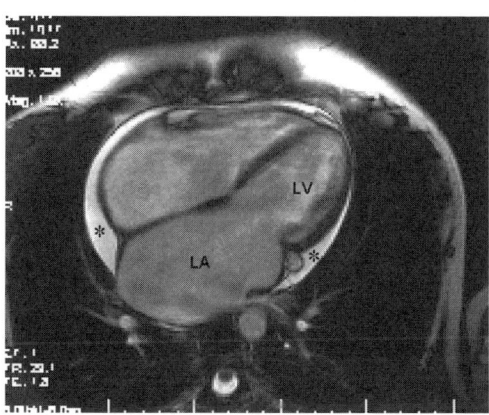

FIGURE 2.27

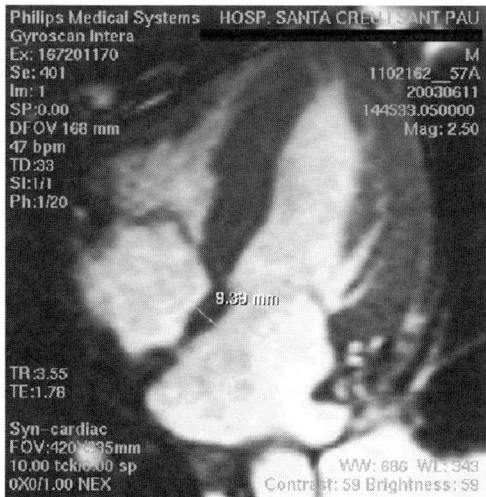

FIGURE 2.28

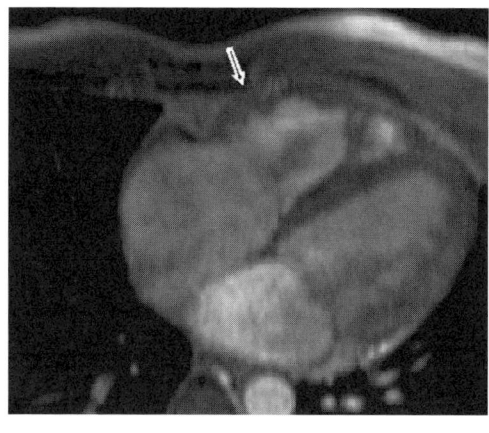

FIGURE 2.29

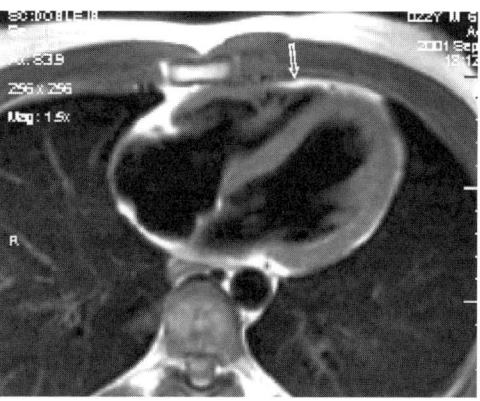

F. 2.25. Delayed contrast enhancement study in a patient with HCM and a previous alcohol ablation. Besides a wedge-shaped area of necrosis at the level of the basal septum (large arrow) secondary to the ablation, a subendocardial septal apical enhancement is also seen (small arrows), with a distribution consistent with a myocardial necrosis in the distal territory of the left anterior descending coronary artery, probably an unwanted effect of the ablation.

F. 2.26. Four-chamber view from a SSFP sequence in a case of primary restrictive cardiomyopathy. Observe the preserved shape of the LV, the absence of apparent hypertrophy, and the dilated atria. A mild pericardial effusion (asterisks) is also present.

F. 2.27. Horizontal long-axis view from a case of cardiac amyloidosis. Note the hypertrophy of the ventricular walls and, also, the interatrial septum.

F. 2.28. GRE axial image in a patient with ARVC showing several small aneurysms of the anterior righ ventricular wall (arrow).

F. 2.29. Axial SE T1w showing an area of fatty infiltration in the anterior right ventricular free wall, which appears thinned and replaced by the adipose tissue.

FIGURE 2.30

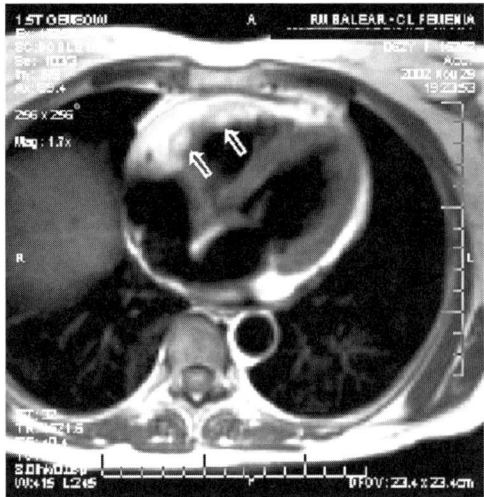 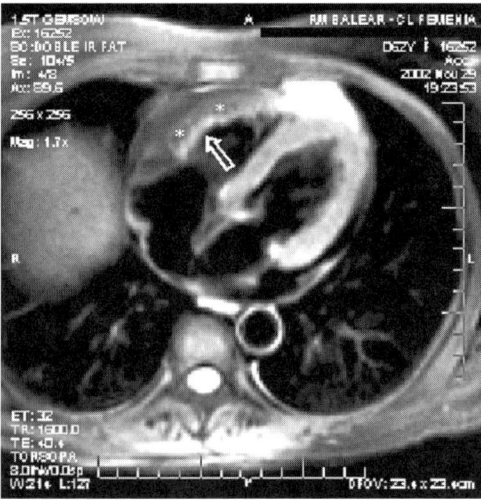

F. 2.30. Fast SE image (left) showing focal high-intensity signals at the right ventricular free wall (arrows) suggestive of fatty infiltration. A fat supressed sequence (right) shows a signal void at these locations (asterisks) confirming the presence of fat; also the thin right ventricular myocardial wall appears now as a structure with intermediate signal intensity (arrow).

ventricular function is preserved in RCM (Cine 2.8 on CD). Cardiac amyloidosis, the most important of secondary forms of RCM, presents with some distinctive features, as is an increased thickness of ventricular and atrial walls, including the interatrial septum (Figure 2.27), some degree of systolic ventricular dysfunction (Cine 2.9 on CD), and a decrease in the myocardial signal intensity, determined as a ratio between myocardium and skeletal muscle, on SE T1w images, this being related to deposition of amyloid protein in the myocardium[36].

CMR is useful, on the other hand, in the differential diagnosis between restrictive cardiomyopathy and constrictive pericarditis. Although some degree of pericardial effusion may be present in RCM, secondary to congestive heart failure, the distinctive finding of a grossly thickened pericardium is highly suggestive of constriction[37] (see chapter on pericardial diseases).

d. Arrhythmogenic right ventricular cardiomyopathy (ARVC)

This genetically transmitted primary form of myocardial disease presents histologically with fibrofatty replacement of the right ventricular myocardium leading to structural and functional alterations of the RV. The diagnosis is based on the presence of a series of major and minor criteria among structural, electrocardiographic, and histological features of the disease[38]. CMR is prefered over other imaging modalities provided its excellent spatial and temporal resolution allowing a detailed study of the RV with cine sequences. Also, the detection of fatty infiltration of the right ventricular wall is possible by means of SE sequences. An imaging protocol including bright- and black-blood sequences encompassing the RV on axial, sagittal and short-axis planes[39] should be obtained in every patient with suspicion of ARVC, as CMR may reveal the presence of some findings considered as major criteria for the diagnosis[40]: 1) significant global dilatation and systolic dysfunction of the RV (Cine 2.10 on CD); 2) localized aneuryms of RV (Figure 2.28); and 3) wall thinning and fatty infiltration (Figure 2.29).

Although fairly sensitive in the diagnosis of ARVC[41], the presence of fat infiltrating the wall of the RV is not a very specific finding[42], and, in fact, a misinterpretation of the normal subepicardial fat as adipose replacement of the right ventricular wall is a frequent cause of false positive diagnoses of ARVC[43]. The obtention of SE and fat-supressed sequences at the same level may be useful in this sense[39] (Figure 2.30). In any case, the assessment of cases with clinical suspicion of ARVC must not rely solely on this finding, but on a complete morphological and functional study of the RV.

References

1. Winterer JT, Lehnhardt S, Schneider B, Neumann K, Allmann KH, Laubenberger J, et al. MRI of heart morphology. Comparison of nongradient echo sequences with single- and multislice acquisition. Invest Radiol 1999; 34: 516–522.

2. Carr JC, Simonetti O, Bundy J, Li D, Pereles S, Finn JP. Cine MR angiography of the heart with segmented true fast imaging with steady-state precession. Radiology 2001; 219: 828–834.

3. Lorenz CH, Walker ES, Morgan VL, Klein SS, Graham TP. Normal human right and left ventricular mass, systolic function, and gender differences by cine magnetic resonance imaging. J Cardiovasc Magn Reson 1999; 1: 7–21.

4. Salton CJ, Chuang ML, O'Donnell CJ, Kupka MJ, Larson MG, Kissinger KV, et al. Gender differences and normal left ventricular anatomy in an adult population free of hypertension. A cardiovascular magnetic resonance study of the Framingham Heart Study Offspring cohort. J Am Coll Cardiol 2002; 39:1055–1060.

5. Miller S, Simonetti OP, Carr J, Kramer U, Finn JP. MR Imaging of the heart with cine True Fast Imaging with Steady-State Precession: influence of spatial and temporal resolutions on left ventricular functional parameters. Radiology 2002; 223: 263–269.

6. Fieno DS, Jaffe WC, Simonetti OP, Judd RM, Finn JP. TrueFISP: assessment of accuracy for measurement of left ventricular mass in an animal model. J Magn Reson Imaging. 2002;15: 526–531.

7. Pons-Lladó G, Carreras F, Borrás X, Llauger J, Palmer J. Echocardiography and Magnetic Resonance Imaging in the assessment of left ventricular mass: a comparative study. Rev Esp Cardiol 2001; 54: 22–28.

8. Myerson SG, Montgomery HE, World MJ, Pennell DJ. Left ventricular mass: reliability of M-mode and 2-dimensional echocardiographic formulas. Hypertension 2002; 40: 673–678.

9. Bellenger NG, Davies LC, Francis JM, Coats AJ, Pennell DJ. Reduction in sample size for studies of remodeling in heart failure by the use of cardiovascular magnetic resonance. J Cardiovasc Magn Reson 2000; 2: 271–278.

10. Marcus JT, DeWaal LK, Götte MJW, van der Geest RJ, Heethaar RM, Van Rossum AC. MRI-derived left ventricular function parameters and mass in healthy young adults: Relation with gender and body size. Int J Card Imaging 1999; 15: 411–419.

11. Sandstede J, Lipke C, Beer M, Hofmann S, Pabst T, Kenn W, et al. Age- and gender-specific differences in left and right ventricular cardiac function and mass determined by cine magnetic resonance imaging. Eur Radiol 2000;10: 438–42.

12. Alfakih K, Plein S, Thiele H, Jones T, Ridgway JP, Sivananthan MU. Normal human left and right ventricular dimensions for MRI as assessed by turbo gradient echo and steady-state free precession imaging sequences. J Magn Reson Imaging. 2003; 17: 323–329.

13. Markievicz W, Sechtem U, Higgins CB. Evaluation of the right ventricle by magnetic resonance imaging. Am Heart J 1987; 113: 8–15.

14. Shors SM, Fung CW, Francois CJ, Finn JP, Fieno DS. Accurate quantification of right ventricular mass at MR imaging by using cine true fast imaging with steady-state precession: study in dogs. Radiology 2004; 230: 383–388.

15. Grothues F, Moon JC, Bellenger NG, Smith GS, Klein HU, Pennell DJ. Interstudy reproducibility of right ventricular volumes, function, and mass with cardiovascular magnetic resonance. Am Heart J 2004; 147: 218–223.

16. Cottin Y, Touzery C, Guy F, Lalande A, Ressencourt O, Roy S, et al. MR imaging of the heart in patients after myocardial infarction: effect of increasing intersection gap on measurements of left ventricular volume, ejection fraction, and wall thickness. Radiology 1999; 213: 513–520.

17. Sievers B, Kirchberg S, Bakan A, Franken U, Trappe HJ. Impact of papillary muscles in ventricular volume and ejection fraction assessment by cardiovascular magnetic resonance. J Cardiovasc Magn Reson 2004; 6: 9–16.

18. Chuang ML, Hibberd MG, Salton CJ, Beaudin RA, Riley MF, Parker RA, et al. Importance of imaging method over imaging modality in noninvasive determination of left ventricular volumes and ejection fraction: assessment by two- and three-dimensional echocardiography and magnetic resonance imaging. J Am Coll Cardiol 2000; 35: 477–484.

44

19. Cerqueira MD, Weissman NJ, Dilsizian V, Jacobs AK, Kaul S, Laskey WK, et al. Standardized myocardial segmentation and nomenclature for tomographic imaging of the heart: a statement for healthcare professionals from the Cardiac Imaging Committee of the Council on Clinical Cardiology of the American Heart Association. Circulation 2002; 105: 539–542.

20. Van der Geest RJ, Buller VG, Jansen E, Lamb HJ, Baur LH, van der Wall EE, et al. Comparison between manual and semiautomated analysis of left ventricular volume parameters from short-axis MR images. J Comput Assist Tomogr 1997; 21: 756–765.

21. Jauhiainen T, Jarvinen VM, Hekali PE, Poutanen VP, Penttila A, Kupari M. MR gradient echo volumetric analysis of human cardiac casts: focus on the right ventricle. J Comput Assist Tomogr 1998; 22: 899–903.

22. Alfakih K, Plein S, Bloomer T, Jones T, Ridgway J, Sivananthan M. Comparison of right ventricular volume measurements between axial and short axis orientation using steady-state free precession magnetic resonance imaging. J Magn Reson Imaging 2003; 18: 25–32.

23. Bellenger NG, Francis JM, Davies CL, Coats AJ, Pennell DJ. Establishment and performance of a magnetic resonance cardiac function clinic. J Cardiovasc Magn Reson 2000; 2: 15–22.

24. Strohm O, Schulz-Menger J, Pilz B, Osterziel KJ, Dietz R, Friedrich MG. Measurement of left ventricular dimensions and function in patients with dilated cardiomyopathy. J Magn Reson Imaging 2001; 13: 367–371.

25. Kim RJ, Wu E, Rafael A, Chen EL, Parker MA, Simonetti O, et al. The use of contrast-enhanced magnetic resonance imaging to identify reversible myocardial dysfunction. N Engl J Med 2000; 343: 1445–1453.

26. Wu E, Judd RM, Vargas JD, Klocke FJ, Bonow RO, Kim RJ. Visualisation of presence, location, and transmural extent of healed Q-wave and non-Q-wave myocardial infarction. Lancet 2001; 357: 21–28.

27. McCrohon JA, Moon JC, Prasad SK, McKenna WJ, Lorenz CH, Coats AJ, et al. Differentiation of heart failure related to dilated cardiomyopathy and coronary artery disease using gadolinium-enhanced cardiovascular magnetic resonance. Circulation 2003; 108: 54–59.

28. Oechslin EN, Attenhofer Jost CH, Rojas JR, Kaufmann PA, Jenni R. Long-term follow-up of 34 adults with isolated left ventricular noncompaction: a distinct cardiomyopathy with poor prognosis. J Am Coll Cardiol 2000; 36: 493–500.

29. Bax JJ, Atsma DE, Lamb HJ, Rebergen SA, Bootsma M, Voogd PJ, et al. Noninvasive and invasive evaluation of noncompaction cardiomyopathy. J Cardiovasc Magn Reson 2002; 4: 353–357.

30. Pons-Lladó G, Carreras F, Borrás X, Llauger J, Palmer J, Bayés de Luna A. Comparison of morphologic assessment of hypertrophic cardiomyopathy by magnetic resonance versus echocardiographic imaging. Am J Cardiol 1997; 79: 1651–1656.

31. Moon JC, Fisher NG, McKenna WJ, Pennell DJ. Detection of apical hypertrophic cardiomyopathy by cardiovascular magnetic resonance in patients with non-diagnostic echocardiography. Heart 2004; 90: 645–649.

32. Choudhury L, Mahrholdt H, Wagner A, Choi KM, Elliott MD, Klocke FJ, et al. Myocardial scarring in asymptomatic or mildly symptomatic patients with hypertrophic cardiomyopathy. J Am Coll Cardiol 2002; 40: 2156–2164.

33. Kim RJ, Judd RM, Gadolinium-enhanced magnetic resonance imaging in hypertrophic cardiomyopathy. J Am Coll Cardiol 2003; 41: 1568–1572.

34. Moon JC, McKenna WJ, McCrohon JA, Elliott PM, Smith GC, Pennell DJ. Toward clinical risk assessment in hypertrophic cardiomyopathy with gadolinium cardiovascular magnetic resonance. J Am Coll Cardiol 2003; 41: 1561–1567.

35. van Dockum WG, ten Cate FJ, ten Berg JM, Beek AM, Twisk JW, Vos J, et al. Myocardial infarction after percutaneous transluminal septal myocardial ablation in hypertrophic obstructive cardiomyopathy: evaluation by contrast-enhanced magnetic resonance imaging. J Am Coll Cardiol 2004; 43: 27–34.

36. Celletti F, Fattori R, Napoli G, Leone O, Rocchi G, Reggiani LB, et al. Assessment of restrictive cardiomyopathy of amyloid or idiopathic etiology by magnetic resonance imaging. Am J Cardiol. 1999; 83: 798–801.

37. Masui T, Finck S, Higgins CB. Constrictive pericarditis and restrictive cardiomyopathy:

evaluation with MR imaging. Radiology 1992; 182: 369–73.

38. McKenna WJ, Thiene G, Nava A, Fontaliran F, Blomstrom-Lundqvist C, Fontaine G, et al. Diagnosis of arrhythmogenic right ventricular dysplasia/cardiomyopathy. Br Heart J 1994; 71: 215–218.

39. Tandri H, Friedrich MG, Calkins H, Bluemke DA. MRI of arrhythmogenic right ventricular cardiomyopathy/dysplasia. J Cardiovasc Magn Reson 2004; 6: 557–563.

40. Pennell DJ. Arrhythmogenic right ventricular cardiomyopathy. Council of the European Society of Cardiology. E-Journal of Cardiology Practice (http://www.escardio.org/knowl-edge/cardiology_practice/ejournal_vol1/Vol1_no7.htm)

41. Tandri H, Calkins H, Nasir K, Bomma C, Castillo E, Rutberg J, et al. Magnetic resonance imaging findings in patients meeting task force criteria for arrhythmogenic right ventricular dysplasia. J Cardiovasc Electrophysiol 2003;14: 476–482.

42. Bluemke DA, Krupinski EA, Ovitt T, Gear K, Unger E, Axel L, et al. MR Imaging of arrhythmogenic right ventricular cardiomyopa-thy: morphologic findings and interobserver reliability. Cardiology 2003; 99:153–162.

43. Bomma C, Rutberg J, Tandri H, Nasir K, Roguin A, Tichnell C, et al. Misdiagnosis of arrhythmogenic right ventricular dysplasia/car-diomyopathy. J Cardiovasc Electrophysiol 2004;15: 300–306.

3

Acquired Diseases of the Aorta

GUILLEM PONS-LLADÓ

As a reliable imaging technique, CMR has a definite role in the study of acquired aortic diseases. Although the information provided by CMR may overlap with that obtained by other imaging methods, it has some important advantages in particular aspects (Table 3.1). From a practical point of view, highlights of CMR are its noninvasive character, the possibility of obtaining planes of the entire aortic length with any orientation, even without contrast agents, its excellent image definition, including the vessel wall, and its comprehensive presentation format.

3.1 Technical Aspects of the Aortic Study by CMR: Imaging the Normal Aorta

Due to the longitudinal position of the vessel in the body, transversal sections can be obtained on thoracic and abdominal axial planes, while along both coronal and sagittal planes the aorta is imaged on its longitudinal view (see chapter 1). However, the orientation of the thoracic aorta requires an oblique sagittal plane if a view including the ascending and descending portion of the vessel is desired (Figure 3.1). Although imaging the aorta by means of two-dimensional methods, either with spin-echo (SE) or gradient-echo (GRE) sequences, provides reliable information on most pathological processes of the vessel, new three-dimensional (3D) angiographic techniques, known as Magnetic Resonance Angiography (MRA), have emerged as a first-line method for studying aortic diseases giving images with high spatial resolution within short acquisition times[1] (Figure 3.2).

An important point when studying the aorta is the measurement of crossectional diameters at different levels of the vessel. While axial or saggital views (Figure 3.1) are useful for measuring diameters of the ascending or decending segments of the aorta, a coronal plane at the level of the aortic valve allows the estimation of diameters of the valve ring and the aortic root (Figure 3.3). A cine sequence obtained by a GRE sequence or, better, using one of the recently introduced steady-state free precession (SSFP) techniques, on this same orientation is useful for the detection of an

Table 3.1 Comparative advantages of different imaging techniques in the study or acquired aortic diseases

	Plain radiograph	Contrast Angiography	CT scanner (multislice)	Echo (thoracic)	Echo (esophageal)	CMR
Noninvasiveness	+	−	+	++	−	++
Field of view	+	+	++	+	+	++
Planes on any orientation	+	+	++	+	+	++
Study of the entire vessel	−	++	++	−	+	++
Resolution without contrast	+	−	+	++	++	++
Dyanamic studies	−	++	+	++	++	++
Flow quantitation	−	++	−	+	+	++
Vessel wall exam	−	+	++	++	++	++
Comprehensible interpretation	−	+	++	+	++	++
Availability and reasonable cost	++	+	++	++	+	+

eventual aortic valve disfunction, due to the direct visualization of blood flow turbulence that these sequences allow, presented as a "signal void" naturally contrasting with with normal laminar blood flow (Cine loop 3.1 on CD).

As mentioned above, currently contrast-enhanced MRA is the method of choice in the routine clinical assessment of vascular disease. By using postprocessing techniques such as maximum intensity projection (MIP) algorithm, a projection image that provides a general overview of the anatomy is obtained (Figure 3.2). These format images are very helpful for clinical evaluation of the vessel morphology and its relationship with other surrounding vascular structures (Cine loop 3.2 on CD). On the other hand, computerized tridimensional reconstruction techniques applied to tomographies of the aorta obtained with paramagnetic contrast, images can be obtained in which the vessel can be imaged as if viewed from within. As the observer can then move at will along the aortic course, the technique has come to be known as virtual aortic endoscopy[2].

3.2 Aortic Aneurysm

The dilatation of a segment of the aorta is a frequent problem, whether it is due to a congenital defect of the connective tissue, as in Marfan's syndrome, or as part of the spectrum of atherosclerosis. CMR has become the technique of choice for the study of aortic aneurysm due to its advantages, already mentioned. Although a contrast-enhanced MRA of the entire thoracic aorta is a fast and very useful technique for the assessment of a segmental dilatation of the aorta (Figure 3.4), simple SE sequences on axial, sagittal or coronal planes also allow a reliable study of an aortic aneurysm, including its localization, extension, and maximal diameter (Figure 3.5). GRE sequences are also useful due to the high signal intensity of flowing blood, that allows the distinction of vascular structures from other, and the detection of thrombus (Figure 3.6).

It is known that the decision to consider aortic aneurysm surgery is based on the value of the maximal diameter of the aortic lumen at the level of the aneurysm. Therefore, it is of particular interest the possibility of performing follow-up studies with exact and reproducible measurements, which may have important implications regarding the timing of surgery (Figure 3.7).

3.3 Aortic Dissection and Related Entities

a. Strategy for the study of aortic dissection by CMR

It is known that clinical data[3] and signs form conventional diagnostic tests[4] have a limited diagnostic accuracy in patients with acute aortic syndrome. Thus, there is a need for a

FIGURE 3.1

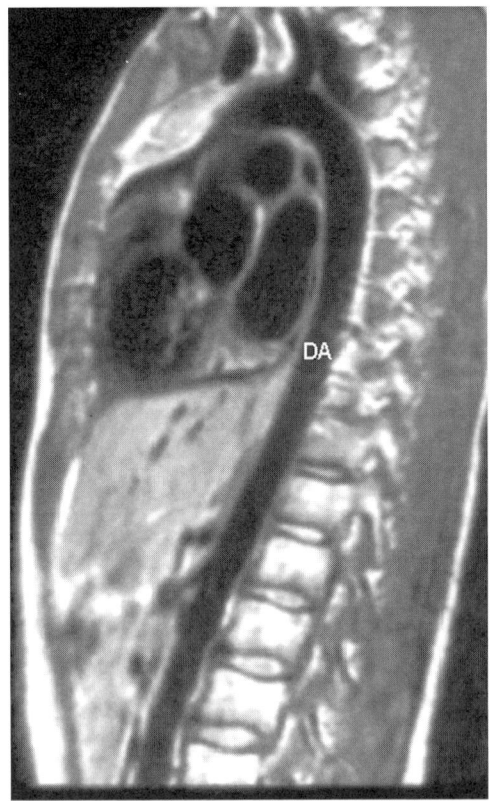

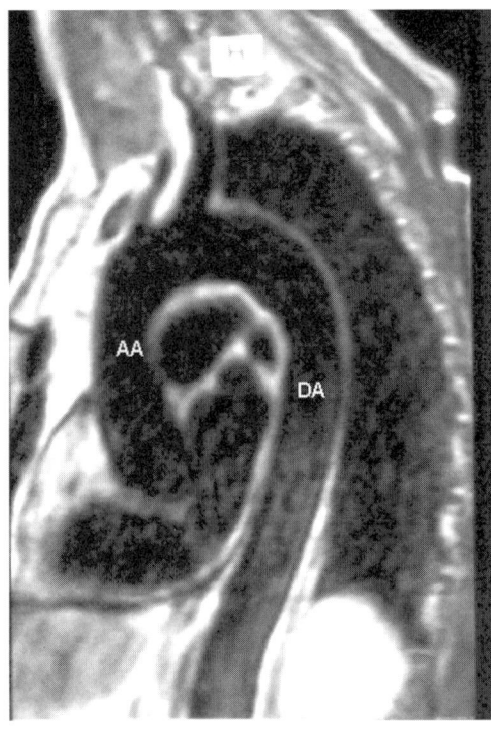

FIGURE 3.2

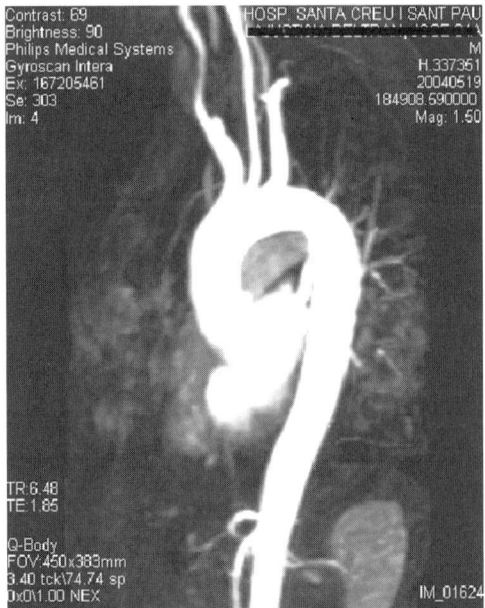

FIGURE 3.3

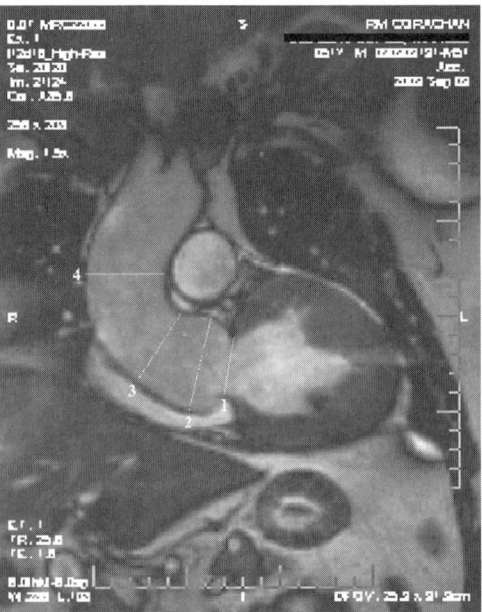

FIGURE 3.4

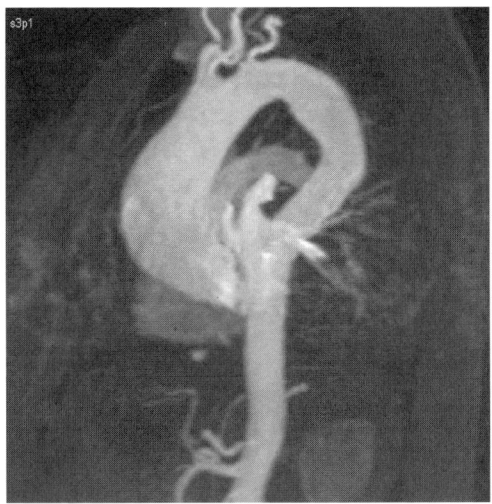

FIGURE 3.5

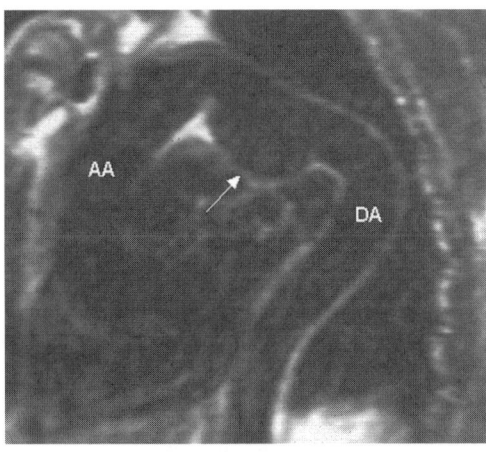 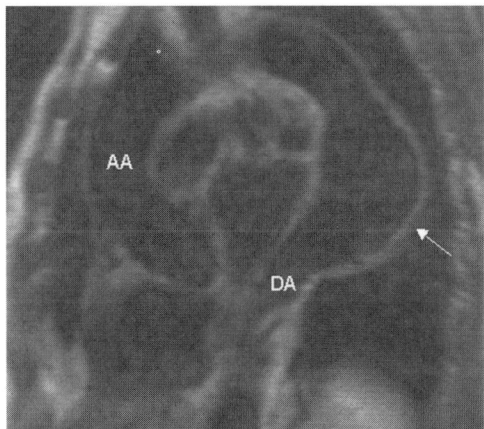

F. 3.1. SE sagittal plane of the normal aorta (left), where only the descending portion of the vessel (DA) is seen; the orientation of the vessel in the body requires a slightly oblique view (right) to encompass also the ascending aorta (AA).

F. 3.2. Maximal intensity projection (MIP) of an MRA of the aorta using a contrast agent.

F. 3.3. Coronal view of an SSFP "bright blood" sequence oriented on the left ventricular outflow tract and the proximal segments of the aorta, where dimensions of the aortic annulus (1), aortic root (2), sino-tubular junction (3), and ascending aorta (4) can be reliably measured.

F. 3.4. 3D reconstruction of an MRI angiography showing ectasia of the aortic root and the ascending aorta, and a tortuous course of the arch and the descending aorta.

F. 3.5. Oblique sagittal views of the thoracic aorta from two different patients encompassing both the ascending (AA) and descending (DA) aorta; a saccular aneurysm (arrow) of the inferior aspect of the aortic arc is seen at left, while a fusiform aneurysm (arrow) of the descending portion of the vessel is displayed at right.

FIGURE 3.6

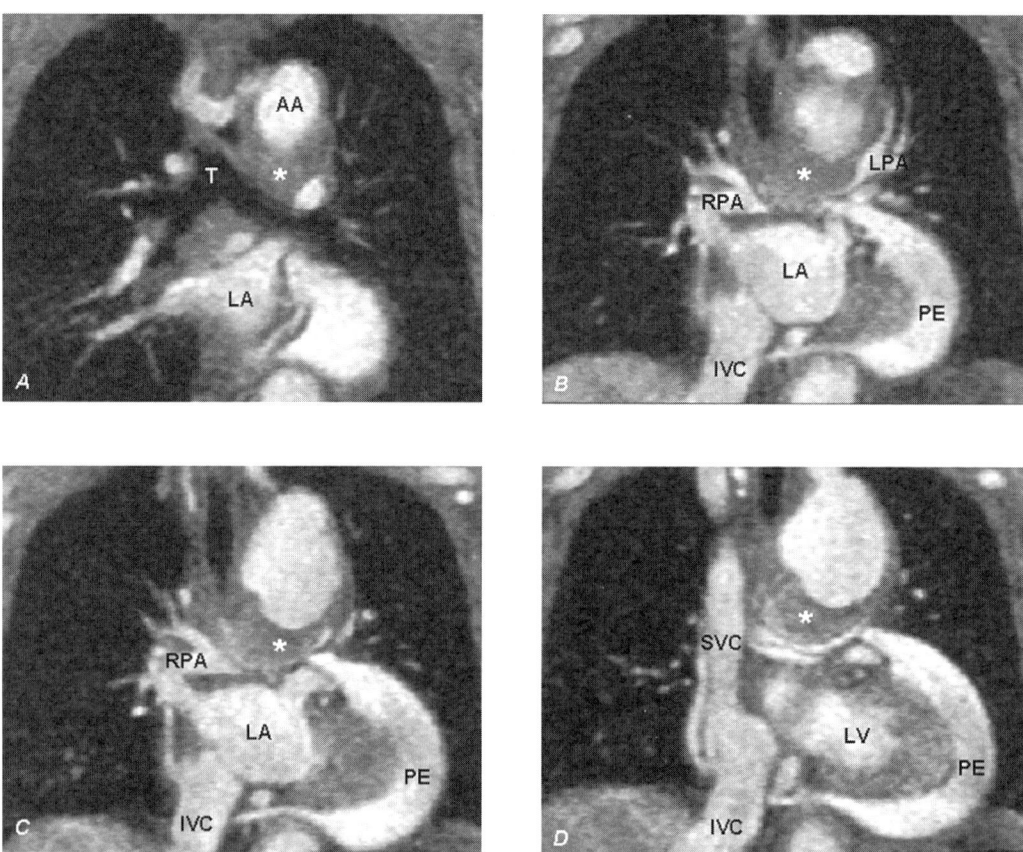

FIGURE 3.7

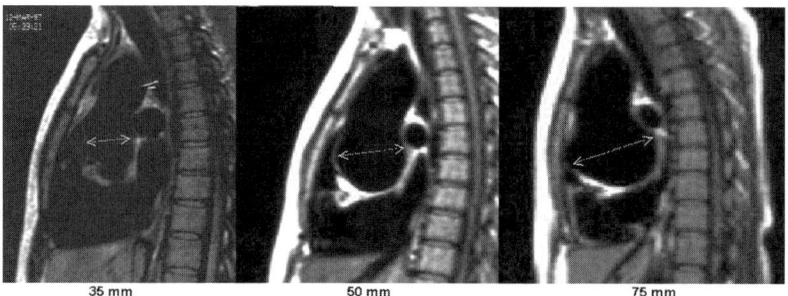

35 mm   50 mm   75 mm

F. 3.6. Parallel coronal views from a Fast-GRE sequence. Planes are selected from back to front (A to D), where a large aneurysm of the aortic arch (AA) is seeen that expands inferiorly, being its inferior aspect occupied by a mural thrombus (asterisks). Note the displacement and compression of both right (RPA) and left (LPA) pulmonary arteries due to the aneurysm. A comprehensive assessment of the different anatomical structures and of its relationship in this case is possible due to the exquisite contrast between flowing blood and stationary tissues. IVC: inferior vena cava; LA: left atrium; LV: left ventricle; PE: pericardial effusion; SVC: superior vena cava; T: trachea.

F. 3.7. Sagittal SE planes taken at yearly intervals from a patient with Takayasu arteritis showing a definite increase in the diameter of the ascending aorta.

reliable imaging technique, CMR being particularly well suited for this purpose[5]. However, a first important aspect to consider when acute aortic dissection is suspected is the clinical situation of the patient. It must be kept in mind that CMR equipment is generally not located near intensive care units and that the study requires about 20–30 minutes to be completed. Also, during this time the immediate access to the patient is restricted, both for patient monitoring and for an eventual emergency medical treatment, although the experience of groups that have performed CMR studies on series of patients with acute dissection has shown that there have not been complications attributable to isolation in any case[6]. Probably due to these aspects, however, computed tomography is still the first choice in the diagnosis of acute dissection, in practice, followed by transesophageal echocardiography, although in a good deal of patients at least two different diagnostic tests have to be performed[7].

When considering CMR for the diagnosis of acute dissection, contrast-enhanced MR angiography is probably the method of choice, as it provides excellent spatial and contrast resolution images in a significantly shorter duration scan than conventional sequences (Figure 3.8). However, a complete study combining the different CMR sequences available is very useful when the clinical situation permits such an strategy, as in chronic dissection[8]. An adequate protocol should include the following sequences:

1. Contrast-enhanced MRA oriented in an oblique sagittal plane along the ascending and descending aorta, obtaining a format image of particular interest since it is the same view than that from conventional contrast aortography, a view which both clinicians and surgeons are familar with (Figure 3.8). This sequence allows the identification of the presence and extension of the intimal membrane, as well as an assessment of flow conditions within the false lumen. There are important technical aspects to consider when planning the obtention of an aortic angiography: one of them is to be sure that the stack covers both the ascending and descending aorta for which we can modify parameters such as slice thickness and number of slices, although an increase in the number of slices prolongs the scan duration and, thus, the length of the breath-hold. Ideally, a breath-hold of less than 20 seconds should be afforded to guarantee patient's collaboration, and a slice thickness between 1.5–2 mm is sufficient for obtaining appropriate images.

2. Thoracic axial T1w SE series

By means of this sequence, transversal images of the thoracic aorta are acquired, ideally from the level of the supra-aortic vessels down to the diafragm. In the case of dissection, the presence of the dissected intimal layer in the aortic lumen can be detected, as well as its extension along the vessel (Figure 3.9). It is also easy to determine the diameters of the different aortic segments. Although the absence of signal in the interior of the false lumen confidently indicates that circulating flow exists at this level, the presence of a relatively intense signal may correspond to either a condition of slow flow or to the presence of thrombosis of the false lumen (Figure 3.10). The comprehensive and sometimes unique information provided by an axial series on T1w SE justifies, in our view, its obtention in most patients with suspected dissection (Figure 3.11).

3. Cine CMR sequence in GRE including the aortic valvular plane

This sequence can be programmed on a coronal plane including the left vetnricular outflow tract, the valvular plane and the aortic root (Cine loop 3.1 on CD). It provides important information on the eventual involvement of the aortic root by the dissection and on valvular function.

4. Cine GRE along a longitudinal axis of the left ventricle

With this series a left ventriculography is obtained that informs on ventricular dimensions and function, and on the eventual presence of pericardial effusion.

5. Axial abdominal spin-echo sequence

Axial SE series might be important in case of suspicion of extension of the dissection into the abdominal aorta (Figure 3.12), by allowing the study of the possible implication of the visceral arterial trunks. It must be kept in mind, though, that the implementation of this series may cause the patient to be repositioned into the scanner in order to obtain new localizing planes, which entails a consequent time delay.

A complete study following the described protocol may easily take an hour, which is not a problem in studies of chronic dissection but may be inconvenient in the acute patient, in whom a contrast-enhanced MRA study can be

FIGURE 3.8

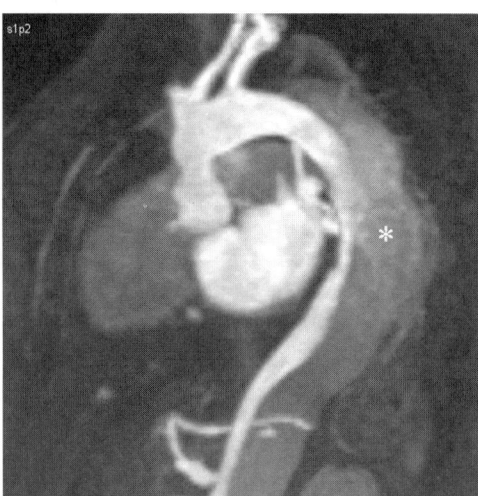

FIGURE 3.10

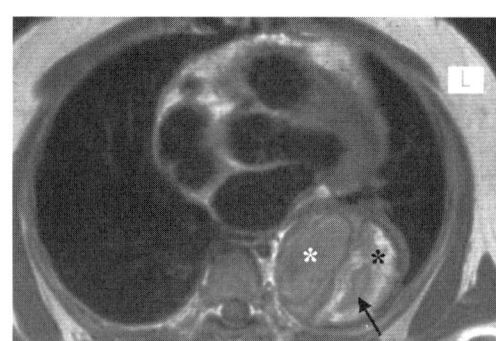

FIGURE 3.9

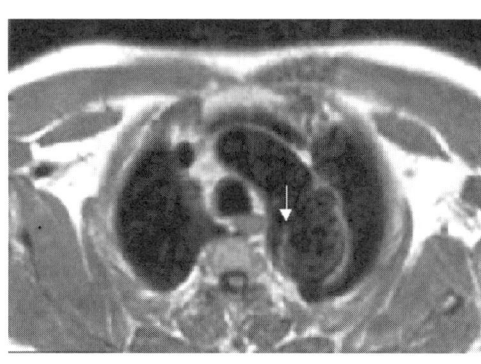

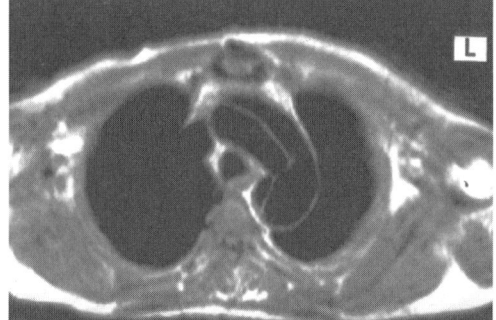

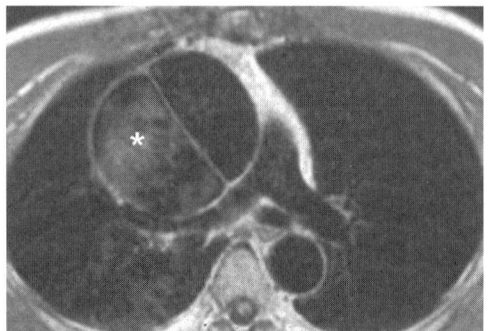

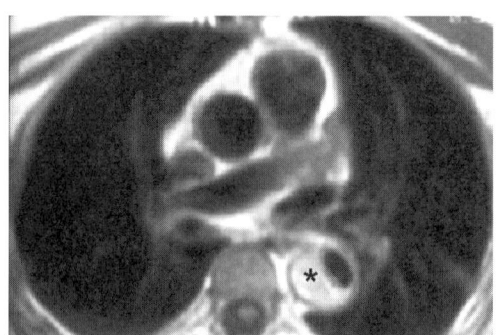

FIGURE 3.11

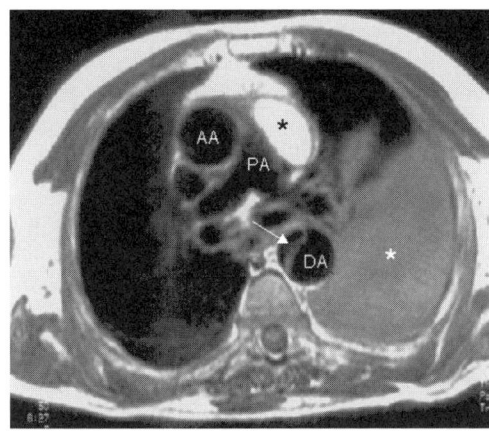 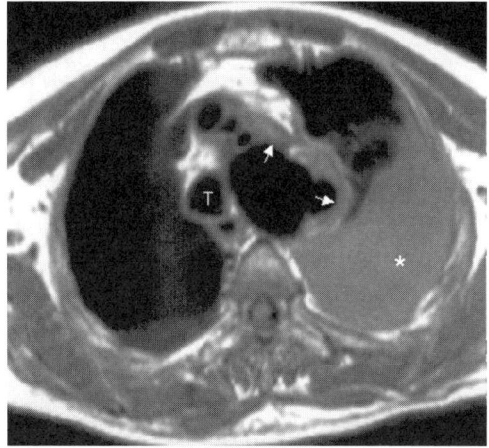

FIGURE 3.12

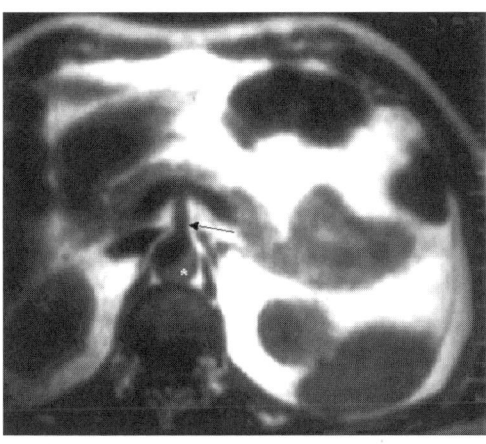

F. 3.8. Maximal intensity projection (MIP) of a contrast MRA study of the aorta in a case of type B dissection showing low signal intensity in the false lumen (asterisk) indicating stagnant flow.

F. 3.9. Axial SE planes in four different patients with aortic dissection. Top left: type B dissection with an entrance tear localized at the aortic arch (arrow); Top right: type A, with the intimo-medial flap visible along the aortic arch, with evidence of flowing blood on both sides of the membrane; Bottom left: type A dissecting aneurysm with a large dilatation of the ascending aorta, where the false channel is detected by the presence of disperse high intensity signals (asterisk) indicating slow flow; Bottom right; type B dissection with uniform highly intense signal in the false lumen (asterisk) suggesting thrombosis of the channel.

F. 3.10. Axial T1w SE image showing dissection in a largely dilated descending aorta; signal intensities from the two lumens are slightly different, from intermediate in the true channel (white arrow), indicating slow flow, to definitely high in the false lumen (black arrow), probably indicating thrombus formation, although with some remaining area of slow flow within (arrow).

F. 3.11. Images from a patient with acute aortic syndrome showing the large amount of key information that the simplest of CMR sequences (i.e.: axial SE) is able to offer. There is a type B dissection, as evidenced by the presence of a flap in the descending aorta (DA) (arrow, on the left panel), with patency at both channels, while the ascending aorta (AA) shows a normal lumen; in addition, there is an aneurismal dilatation of the aortic arch (right panel) that displaces the trachea (T) to the right, and with an increase in the vessel wall thickness (arrows, on the right panel) suggesting intramural hematoma; the exam of the rest of the thorax shows an image of mediastinal hematoma (black asterisk, on the right panel), that compresses the pulmonary artery (PA), and is probably very recent, provided its high signal intensity, and an extense left pleural effusion (white asterisks, on both panels).

F. 3.12. SE axial plane at the abdominal level showing aortic dissection with thrombosed false lumen (asterisk); the origin of the superior mesenteric artery (arrow) is visualized arising from the true aortic lumen.

sufficient to obtain a good assessment of the type and the extension of the dissection.

b. Differential diagnosis of aortic dissection by CMR

Since the cornerstone of the diagnosis of aortic dissection is the detection of the dissected intimal-medial membrane, it is important to be aware of some of the possible sources of uncertainty concerning its recognition using CMR. On one hand, there are normal anatomic structures or even artifacts that can lead to a false-positive diagnosis[9]. The images which most frequently have caused confusion in CMR studies are those depicting the left venous brachiocephalic trunk, which runs in close relation to the anterior aspect of the aortic arch, or those showing the posterior aortic pericardium recess (Figure 3.13). These potential causes of confusion appear in T1w SE sequences on axial planes, and do not pose great difficulties, since the possibility of comparing slices at different levels permits its easy recognition provided a certain degree of experience. Obviously, these limitations do not affect studies with the technique of MRA.

On the other hand, there are pathological processes of the aortic wall formerly considered as atypical forms of dissection[10], as an intramural hematoma or a penetrating atherosclerotic ulcer, that today are grouped, together with classical dissection, aneurysm leak and rupture, and traumatic aortic transection, under the term of acute aortic syndrome[11]. These entities must be taken into account in patients with suspected dissection, as its presence also implies a serious prognosis but, due to the lack of a ruptured intimal layer and two lumens into the aorta, may eventually lead to a false negative diagnosis of acute aortic wall disease. Intramural hematoma, or "dissection without rupture" occurs in up to 13% of the cases of dissection, as has been demonstrated in autopsy studies[12]. In these cases, a thickening of the aortic wall of crescent shape or circumferential form has been observed which does not generally deform the circular shape of the aortic lumen. It displays a signal of intermediate intensity which corresponds to the parietal hematoma (Figure 3.14). This type of image must be distinguished from other pathological forms, specifically from a true dissection with thrombosis of the false lumen, which usually displays deformation of the aortic lumen (Figures 3.9 and 3.12). The distinction must be made as well from an atherosclerotic aneurysm with mural thrombosis in its interior, in which an important dilatation of the aorta is present (Figure 3.6). In these cases the information provided by other imaging techniques, such as echocardiography or CT, may be useful, basically by detecting the presence of calcium in the inner wall of the hematoma, that identifies this wall as the true intimo-medial layer of the aorta.

Recognition of the aortic intramural hematoma is of great importance, since it has the same clinical implications than dissection at the acute phase, its evolution in the chronic state being most frequently towards an aortic aneurysm, although complete regression is not infrequent, as is the transformation into a classical dissection[13] (Figure 3.15). These evolutive patterns are not surprising provided the pathophysiology of intramural hematoma[14], where the initial phenomenon is an hemorrhage of the vasa vasorum in the media of the vessel without a rupture of the intimo-medial membrane or, at least, without a re-entry tear, rupture that may occur, however, later in time.

Penetrating atherosclerotic ulcer has a pathogenetic mechanism different from dissection or intramural hematoma[12,14]. In this case it is not a process of degeneration of the media of the artery, but rather a continuous erosion of an atherosclerotic plaque that penetrates beyond the limits of the internal elastic membrane, which may form a localized hematoma and progress toward the formation of a pseudoaneurysm o even an aortic parietal rupture. Its atherosclerotic origin conditions its presentation in elderly patients, normally in the descending aorta. Aortic penetrating ulcer is relatively infrequent, its clinical presentation is variable, not rarely silent, and its fors of evolution is diverse[15]. At CMR, ulcers appear as a focal irregularity of the aortic wall, with an outpouching, or crater, frequently surrounded by an intramural hematoma (Figure 3.16).

These different morphological forms of acute aortic disease may coexist in an individual patient, being in these cases where the comprehensive exam allowed by CMR proves to be the most useful (Figure 3.11).

Rupture of the aorta due to a blunt chest trauma presents with distinctive features that are reliably depicted by imaging techniques[16]. The

FIGURE 3.13

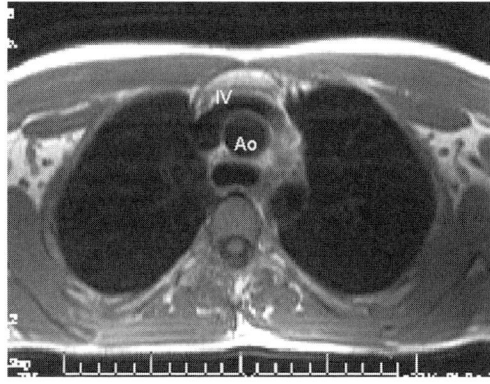
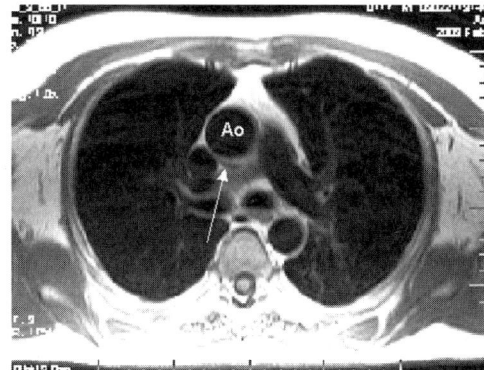

FIGURE 3.14

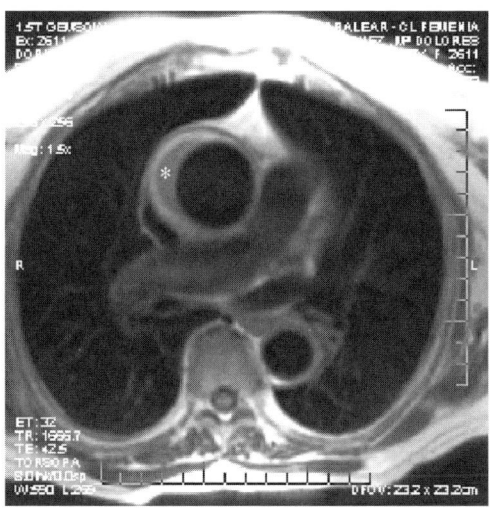

F. 3.13. Axial T1w SE images showing, on the left, the uppermost part of the ascending aorta (Ao) in close relationship with the innominate vein (IV); on the right panel, the posterior aortic pericardial recess (arrow) is seen adjacent to the wall of the ascending aorta.

F. 3.14. Axial "black-blood" sequence in a case of intramural hematoma of the ascending aorta; note the asymmetric, crescent-shaped increase in the aortic wall thickness, with high signal intensity (asterisk).

F. 3.15. Axial SE images from a patient who presented with an image of intramural hematoma of the abdominal aorta (arrow, on the left panel) that progressed to overt dissection one year later (arrow, on the right panel).

FIGURE 3.15

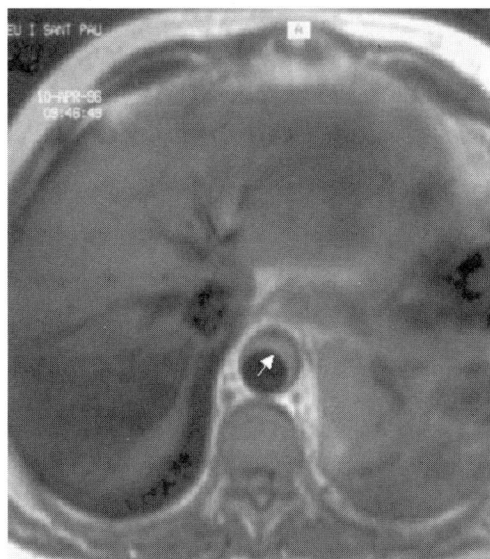
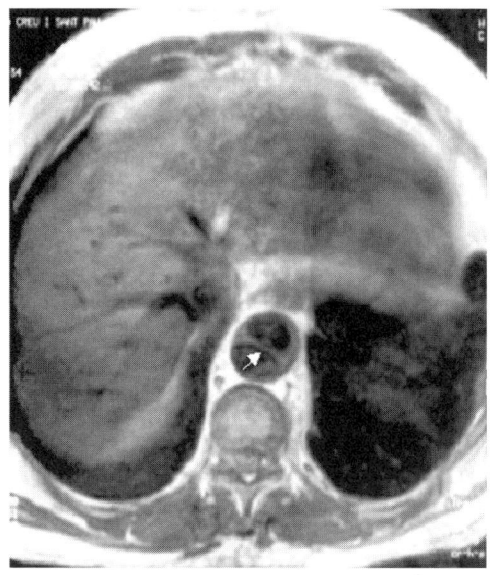

FIGURE 3.16

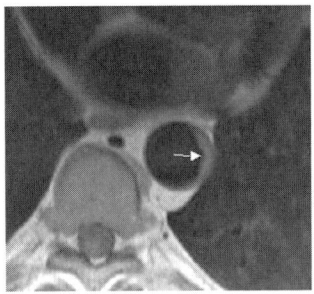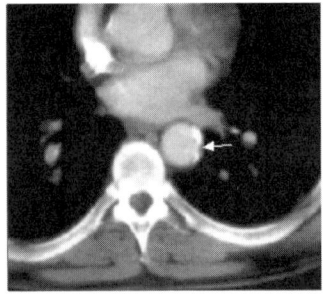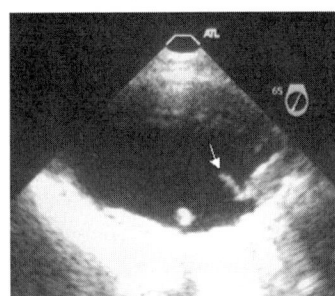

FIGURE 3.17

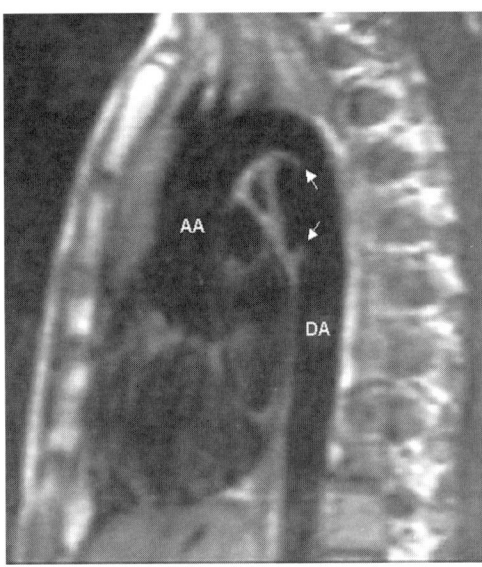

FIGURE 3.18

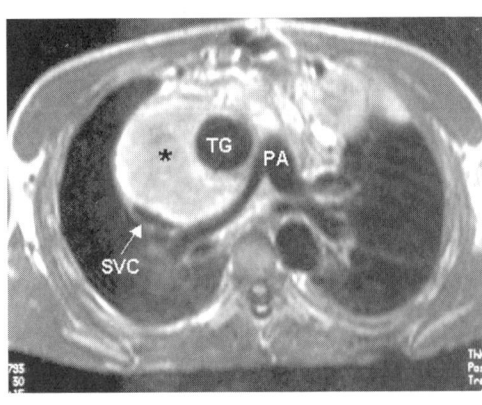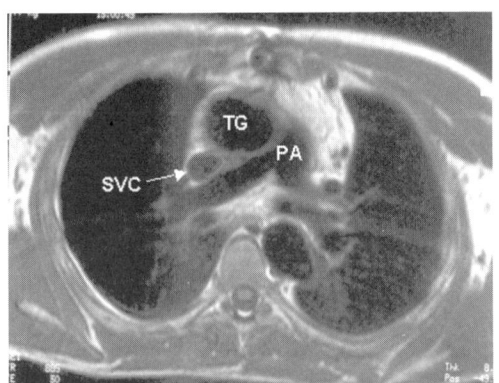

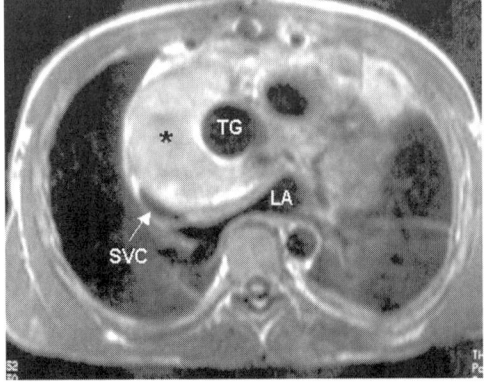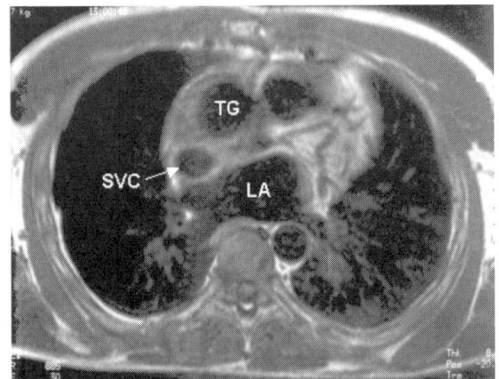

FIGURE 3.19

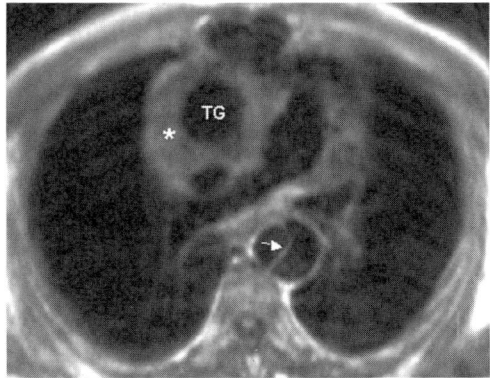 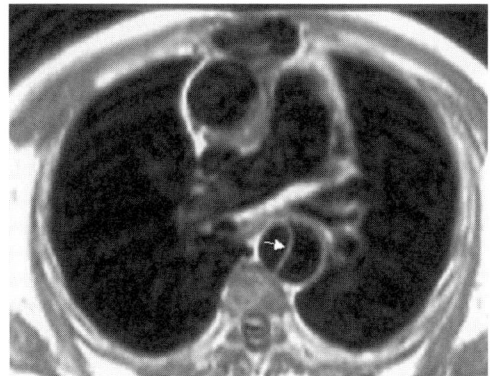

FIGURE 3.20

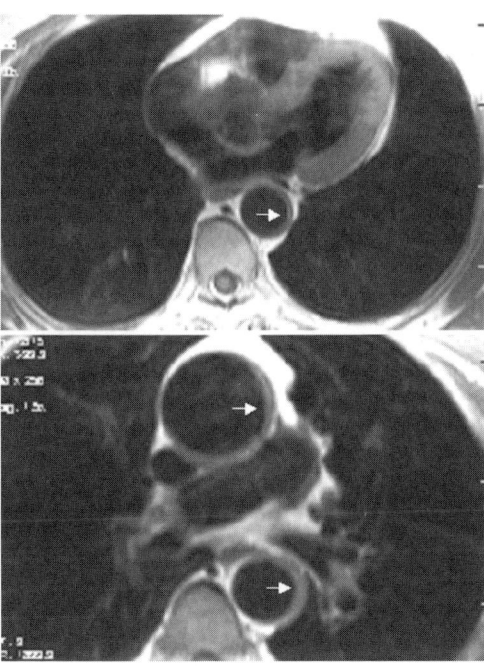

F. 3.16. Contribution of different imaging techniques to the study of penetrating atherosclerotic ulcer. On the left panel, axial image from a CMR "black-blood" sequence showing a localized, medium signal intensity increase in the lateral aortic wall protruding into the lumen with a crater-like indentation (arrow); a CT scanner (middle panel) proved this image to be an atherosclerotic plaque as evidenced by its high calcium contents (arrow); a transeophageal echocardiography (right panel) revealed a localized rupture of the endoluminal layer of this plaque (arrow) proving its ulcerative character.

F. 3.17. Oblique sagittal T1w SE view in a case of traumatic rupture of the aorta: the tears of the intimal layer are visible at the proximal descending aorta (arrows). This exam was obtained years after the patient suffered a serious car crash, the aortic rupture having pass unnoticed since then.

F. 3.18. Axial T1w SE planes obtained on the immediate postoperative state (left panels), and one year after (right ones) in a patient in whom a tubular graft (TG) was placed on the ascending aorta due to a type A dissection. A large peritubular hematoma is seen postoperatively (asterisks, on the left), contained by the native aortic wall that is left wrapped around the graft, and compressing surrounding structures, such as the left atrium (LA), pulmonary artery (PA), and the superior vena cava (SVC). At follow-up, and without any intervention, resorption of the hematoma is evident; note the normal shape appearance of the formerly compressed structures.

F. 3.19. Axial T1w SE planes from a patient operated for type A dissection that extended throughout the descending aorta; a tubular graft (TG) was inserted at the ascending aorta. On the left, the postoperative study shows a moderate peritubular hematoma (asterisk), and a persistence of the membrane of dissection at the descending aorta (arrow). An exam obtained one year after (righ panel) shows disappearance of the hematoma, but persistence of dissection (arrow), even with patency at both lumens. This is a frequent finding late after this kind of intervention.

F. 3.20. Axial T1w SE planes showing increase in the aortic wall due to the presence of atherosclerotic plaques (arrows); note the uniform signal intensity and smooth edge of the lesions.

proximal segment of the descending aorta is the weakest point in case of sudden deceleration of the body and, when not leading to death due to complete rupture, a pseudoaneurysm is formed at this level, with local tearing of the intimo-medial layer and contention of the aortic blood flow by the adventitia (Figure 3.17). This pseudoaneurysm usually has a limited extension, and may pass unnoticed until an appropriate imaging technique is performed.

c. Post-operative or follow-up studies

All patients who survive to an episode of acute aortic syndrome are cause of clinical concern afterwards, wheter an intervention has been performed or not. CMR is an excellent method for these follow-up studies, that require the highest reproducibility.

While a potential evolutive pattern of a particular form of aortic wall disease may be detected over time in unoperated patients (Figure 3.15), postoperative studies may show findings that are important to know (Figure 3.18 and 3.19).

3.4 Study of the atherosclerotic plaque by CMR

On the basis that measurements of arterial wall thickness have proven useful in predicting cardiovascular risk, and provided that CMR is able to image accurately the thoracic aorta, the technique has been applied on large groups of population[17] showing that CMR measurements are highly reproducible, and that aortic wall thickness varies by age, race and sex. The reliable detection of aortic plaque by CMR (Figure 3.20) has prompted studies[18] where it has been shown that the technique can detect aortic atherosclerosis and monitor its evolution over time.

References

1. Tatli S, Lipton MJ, Davison BD, Skorstad RB, Yucel EK. From the RSNA refresher courses: MR imaging of aortic and peripheral vascular disease. Radiographics 2003; 23 (Spec No): S59–78.

2. Vogt FM, Goyen M, Debatin JF. MR angiography of the chest. Radiol Clin North Am. 2003 Jan;41(1):29–41.

3. Armstrong WF, Bach DS, Carey LM, Froehlich J, Lowell M, Kazerooni EA. Clinical and echocardiographic findings in patients with suspected acute aortic dissection. Am Heart J 1998; 136: 1051–1060.

4. von Kodolitsch Y, Nienaber CA, Dieckmann C, Schwartz AG, Hofmann T, Brekenfeld C, et al. Chest radiography for the diagnosis of acute aortic syndrome. Am J Med. 2004; 116: 73–77.

5. Fattori R, Nienaber CA. MRI of acute and chronic aortic pathology: pre-operative and postoperative evaluation. J Magn Reson Imaging 1999; 10: 741–750.

6. Nienaber CA, von Kodolitsch Y, Nicolas V, Siglow V, Piepho A, Brockhoff C, et al. The diagnosis of thoracic aortic dissection by non-invasive imaging procedures. N Engl J Med 1993; 328: 1–9.

7. Moore AG, Eagle KA, Bruckman D, Moon BS, Malouf JS, Fattori R, et al. Choice of computed tomography, transesophageal echocardiography, magnetic resonance imaging, and aortography in acute aortic dissection: International Registry of Acute Aortic Dissection (IRAD). Am J Cardiol 2002; 89: 1235–1238.

8. Kunz RP, Oberholzer K, Kuroczynski W, Horstick G, Krummenauer F, Thelen M, ET AL. Assessment of chronic aortic dissection: contribution of different ECG-gated breath-hold MRI techniques. AJR Am J Roentgenol 2004; 182: 1319–26.

9. Solomon SL, Brown JL, Glazer HS, Mirowitz SA, Lee JKT. Thoracic aortic dissection: pitfalls and artifacts in MR imaging. Radiology 1990; 177: 223–228.

10. Wolff KA, Herold CJ, Tempany CM, Parravano JG, Zerhouni EA. Aortic dissection: atypical patterns seen at MR imaging. Radiology 1991; 181: 489–495.

11. Macura KJ, Corl FM, Fishman EK, Bluemke DA. Pathogenesis in acute aortic syndromes: aortic dissection, intramural hematoma, and penetrating atherosclerotic aortic ulcer. AJR Am J Roentgenol. 2003; 181: 309–16.

12. Wilson SK, Hutchins GM. Aortic dissecting aneurysms: causative factors in 204 subjects. Arch Pathol Lab Med 1982; 106: 175–180

13. Evangelista A, Dominguez R, Sebastia C, Salas A, Permanyer-Miralda G, Avegliano G, et al. Long-term follow-up of aortic intramural hematoma: predictors of outcome. Circulation. 2003; 108: 583–589.

14. Vilacosta I, San Roman JA. Acute aortic syndrome. Heart 2001; 85: 365–368.

15. Cho KR, Stanson AW, Potter DD, Cherry KJ, Schaff HV, Sundt TM 3rd. Penetrating atherosclerotic ulcer of the descending thoracic aorta and arch. J Thorac Cardiovasc Surg 2004; 127: 1393–1399.

16. Fishman JE. Imaging of blunt aortic and great vessel trauma. J Thorac Imaging 2000; 15: 97–103.

17. Li AE, Kamel I, Rando F, Anderson M, Kumbasar B, Lima JA, et al. Using MRI to assess aortic wall thickness in the multiethnic study of atherosclerosis: distribution by race, sex, and age. AJR Am J Roentgenol. 2004; 182: 593–597.

18. Mohiaddin RH, Burman ED, Prasad SK, Varghese A, Tan RS, Collins SA, et al. Glagov remodeling of the atherosclerotic aorta demonstrated by cardiovascular magnetic resonance: the CORDA asymptomatic subject plaque assessment research (CASPAR) project. J Cardiovasc Magn Reson 2004; 6: 517–25.

Study of Valvular Heart Disease

4

LUÍS J. JIMÉNEZ-BORREGUERO

4.1 Introduction

Cardiovascular magnetic resonance (CMR) has proven to be of considerable value in the study of valvular heart disease by assessing its severity, associated complications and its hemodynamic consequences. Although echocardiography continues to be the simplest and most available method in this sense, CMR is an alternative when echocardiographic results are inconclusive or limited. In addition, CMR may be considered a reference method in some aspects of valvular heart disease, as in the calculation of regurgitant volume and fraction in the case of valvular insufficiency[1].

The severity of valvular disease can be evaluated by CMR by means of several methods analyzing not only blood flow behavior but also the hemodynamic consequences of valvular dysfunction. Cine-MR sequences generate images where the phenomena of high flow velocity and turbulence, which characterize stenosis and valvular regurgitation, can be evidenced. Cine loop display of images obtained during different phases of the cardiac cycle provide a dynamic representation of flow behavior in systole and diastole. Physiological laminar flow causes an intense bright signal which highly contrasts with statical structures on the images. High velocity or turbulent flow produced by stenosis or regurgitation presents as a signal void appearing as black or dark grey areas within the normal flow. The intensity and extension of the signal of blood turbulence depends on the technical parameters selected, among which echo time (TE) and spatial resolution stand out. Sequences with long TE are sensitive to turbulences generated by low velocity flows and are, therefore, useful for the study of venous flow. Those with short TE are sensitive to turbulence generated by flow on the high velocity ranges and are used for the analysis of valvular stenosis or regurgitation. Steady state free precession (SSFP) sequences have proved to provide better signal to noise ratio than conventional sequences and improved anatomical resolution of the valves[2, 3] (Figure 4.1 and Cine Loop 4.01 on CD) and ventricles[4].

4.2 Velocity Calculation and Flow Quantitation

With velocity-encoded cine MR imaging, quantitative velocity maps can be obtained in three spatial directions and with the desired orientation without window restrictions and within a wide range of flow velocity values. Currently, CMR sequences most widely used for this purpose are known as phase-contrast images, and are based on the principle that the movement of any structure containing hydrogen generates a phase shift of the radiofrequency waves in the presence of a specific sequence of magnetic gradients and stimuli. The dephasing of the radiofrequency waves is directly proportional to the velocity of the structure or fluid under study. The obtained maps represent in dark grey the velocity of flow in one direction (e.g. caudo-cranial) and in white or bright tones the movement in the opposite direction (e.g. cranio-caudal) (Figure 4.2). As is the case with the other sequences, the cine velocity maps are also obtained from a specific number of cardiac cycles.

In valvular stenosis, flow can be imaged by applying cine MR velocity mapping in multiple contiguous slices parallel to the valvular plane in the receiving cardiac chamber. Velocity is encoded in a direction perpendicular to the study plane in such a way that in some of the selected slices the peak velocity value will be obtained. This occurs in the *vena contracta* region, that is observed within a few millimeters above the valvular planes, where peak velocity values are found (Figure 4.3).

Maximal velocity flow can be also imaged in planes aligned with the stenotic flow (Figure 4.4). In order to avoid underestimation of the recorded velocity, it is recommended that the encoded velocity direction coincide with that of the stenotic jet. Previous representation of flow turbulence with cine gradient-echo images allows a reference for an accurate alignment of the cine velocity maps.

Velocity encoded through the imaging plane, on a crossectional slice of the great arteries or veins, is needed for the calculation of flow volume and rate. The average velocity of the flow in the lumen of the vessel, multiplied by the area of its section, gives a precise calculation of the instantaneous flow[5]. The flow value obtained in each phase of the cardiac cycle is registered on a graph of flow plotted against time (Figure 4.2c and 4.5) the area under the curve representing the flow volume. Besides the quantitative estimation of velocity and flow values, the presentation in cine format of the images provides dynamic information on flow (Cine Loop 4.02 on CD).

4.3 Anatomic Evaluation

The appropriate clinical management of valvular heart disease requires information not only on the clinical situation of the patient and the severity of the valve lesion but also on its hemodynamic consequences on ventricular dimensions and function. Currently, CMR is considered the most accurate method for the assessment of size, thickness and contractile ventricular function[6].

Direct planimetry of the valve area by CMR (Figure 4.3) in cases of aortic valve stenosis was demonstrated to be feasible with GRE sequences[7]. However, SSFP sequences have significantly improved image resolution and reduced flow artifacts, this allowing a more accurate direct planimetry of aortic valve area[2, 3]. Also, valvular leaflets can be examined in motion using cine-MR sequences and the degree of valve thickening can be determined (Figures 4.1). Highly fibrous areas appear in black or dark grey as a consequence of the low signal intensity produced by the fibrous tissue. However, CMR could not differentiate the presence of calcium from fibrosis due to the fact that both generate a similar signal void.

Although transesophageal echocardiography remains the first-choice diagnostic tool for the study of endocarditis, CMR has also been used to demonstrate endocardic vegetations and their complications, such as pseudoaneurysms or abscesses[8, 9]. Endocardial vegetations are identified in cine-MR images as low signal areas in the valvular leaflet. Distinction between flow turbulence secondary to valvular stenosis or insufficiency and that showing a vegetation, can be done by analyzing its movement throughout the cardiac cycle. Whereas that due to stenosis or regurgitation only appear in systole or diastole, respectively, vegetations persists during the entire cardiac

62

FIGURE 4.1

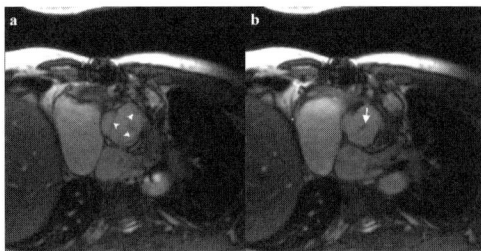

FIGURE 4.4

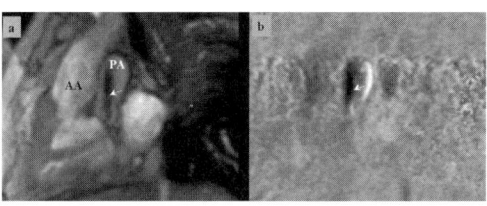

FIGURE 4.2

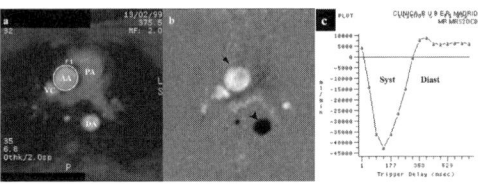

FIGURE 4.3

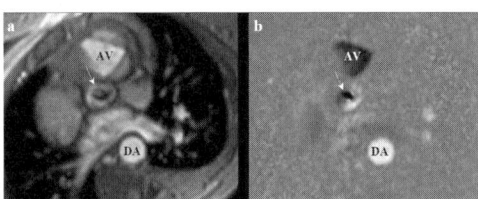

FIGURE 4.5

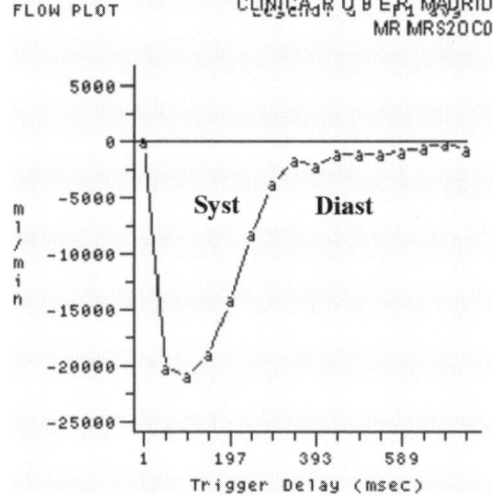

F. 4.1. Mild aortic regurgitation. Systolic (a) and diastolic (b) frames of a cine SSFP sequence on the aortic valve plane. In the systolic image three aortic leaflets (head arrows) are evident. In the diastolic frame the signal void (arrow) corresponds to the orifice of the aortic valve insufficiency defect.

F. 4.2. Severe aortic regurgitation. Cine phase contrast diastolic frame of an axial plane of the ascending aorta (AA), upper vena cava (VC) and descending aorta (DA). A) Magnitude image allows the anatomical measurement of the crossectional area of the aorta. B) Velocity map with velocity encoded through plane, allowing the measurement of the mean velocity through the aorta (arrow); bright and dark intensity signal within vascular structures depend on the velocity and direction of flow: compare signals within the ascending (arrow) and the descending (arrow head) aorta. C) Flow-velocity curve in the ascending aorta: observe the regurgitant diastolic flow that can be quantified and related to systolic flow to calculate regurgitant fraction.

F. 4.3. Crossectional plane of the aortic and pulmonary valves in a patient with great vessels transposition. A): Magnitude systolic frame of a cine phase contrast sequence in a plane perpendicular to the flow direction showing that the aortic valve (AV) has three leaflets and the pulmonary valve is highly stenotic with a planimetry estimated area of 0.5 cm2 (arrow). B): Systolic frame of a velocity map with velocity encoded through plane direction showing high velocity flow at the level of the pulmonary valve (arrow). DA: descending aorta.

F. 4.4. A) Magnitude systolic frame of a cine phase-contrast sequence in a plane with same direction than the systolic jet of the pulmonary valve stenosis. B) Velocity map with velocity encoded in same direction than the jet shows high velocity flow at the level of the *vena contracta* (arrow).

F. 4.5. Normal flow curve in the ascending aorta: compare with a curve in the case of an aortic regurgitation, as shown in Figure 4.2c.

cycle. In those rare cases in which echocardiography is inconclusive CMR may be an alternative for the diagnosis and evaluation of valvular endocarditis and its complications.

4.4 Aortic Regurgitation

a. Quantitation with cine velocity mapping

Calculation of the regurgitant volume or fraction permits precise quantitation of the severity of valvular aortic insufficiency: the velocity is encoded through plane so that the flow velocity over the entire surface of the aortic section can be analyzed (Figure 4.2). It is important to be sure that the study plane is strictly orthogonal to the ascending aorta, immediately distal to the level of the aortic root (Figure 4.6). Unlike Doppler echocardiography, which samples blood velocity in a small volume, phase-contrast cine MR simultaneously analyzes flow over the entire cross-ection of the aorta. This advantage permits a precise calculation of the flow volume in each phase of the cardiac cycle, which is obtained by multiplying the average velocity by the area of the section. The planimetry of the area under the diastolic curve of retrograde flow represents the aortic regurgitation volume (Figure 4.2c). The regurgitant fraction is obtained by dividing retrograde diastolic flow volume by the normal antegrade systolic flow.

In the phase contrast image, the normal flow in the ascending aorta is presented in intense white or black tones (depending on the encoding map), while the absence of a retrograde flow in diastole causes a lack of a definite flow signal (Cine Loop 4.2 on CD). Aortic valvular insufficiency produces retrograde aortic flow that is recorded in a tone opposite to that of the anterograde flow in the ascending aorta (Cine Loop 4.3 on CD).

b. Quantitation of regurgitant volume using Simpson's method

Ventricular volumes can be calculated by series of slices covering the entire ventricular chambers[6] (Figure 4.7) (see Chapter 2). From the obtained diastolic and systolic right and left ventricular volumes, the stroke volume (SV) of each ventricle is calculated. Provided the presence on an aortic regurgitation, and the absence of any other significant valvular insufficiency, or shunt, the quantitation of the regurgitant fraction can be performed by comparison of the stroke volume of the left and right ventricles ([LVSV-RVSV]/LVSV), where LVSV is stroke volume of the left ventricle, RVSV is the stroke volume of the right ventricle and LVSV-RVSV equals the volume of aortic regurgitation. This is an accurate method to quantify aortic regurgitation[10, 11].

c. Evaluation of regurgitation with cine gradient-echo

By this method, images of the outflow tract of the left ventricle and the ascending aorta in coronal planes of the thorax are obtained. Turbulence and high flow velocity of the regurgitant jet appear in GRE images as an area of signal void that highly contrasts with the normal flow into the left ventricular chamber. By analyzing the area of signal void, an estimation of the severity of aortic regurgitation may be done[12]. The width, depth, and the area or the volume of the turbulent regurgitation jet are related to regurgitation severity similarly to the current echocardiographic color flow map techniques. However, it has to be noted that this does not apply to newer fast-GRE sequences such as SSFP, which due to a lower TE may lead to an underestimation of the regurgitant flow.

The acceleration of flow proximal to the regurgitant leak produces a diastolic signal void near the aortic side of the valve (Figure 4.8). Its size correlates with the grade of aortic regurgitation[13]. Another quantitative approach to this method by velocity mapping has been proposed[14].

4.5 Mitral and Tricuspid Regurgitation

a. Quantitation with cine velocity mapping

Mitral insufficiency can be quantitated with this technique by calculation of flow volume in the mitral ring and ascending aorta[15]. The difference between left ventricular inflow volume and aortic flow volume, and the regurgitant fraction can be calculated in order to estimate the severity of mitral regurgitation.

Another approach to qualitative estimation of tricuspid insufficiency is based on the study of flow the vena cava. The flow of the superior vena cava can also be estimated on the same plane used to analyze the aorta. Flow can be calculated from data obtained from velocity maps by multiplying the area of the vena cava section during each cardiac cycle by its velocity. In normal subjects, a systolic and a diastolic wave toward the right atrium and another retrograde diastolic wave that coincides with atrial contraction are observed[16]. Patients with significant tricuspid regurgitation display a flat or inverted systolic wave.

b. Quantitation of regurgitant volume using Simpson's method

Volume calculation is carried out using the same method as the one described for aortic regurgitacion. Quantitation of the regurgitant fraction is obtained by comparing the stroke volume of the left and right ventricles ([LVSV-RVSV]/LVSV, where LVSV-RVSV equals the mitral regurgitant volume. This parameter has proved to have an excellent correlation with the severity of mitral insufficiency, as long as no other significant regurgitations or shunts are present[10, 11]. The same procedure is used for tricuspid insufficiency ([RVSV-LVSV]/RVSV), where RVSV-LVSV is the tricuspid regurgitant volume.

c. Evaluation with cine gradient echo

Oblique planes including the longitudinal axis of the left ventricle are preferred to visualize the origin of systolic turbulence of mitral regurgitation. Volume, depth and the area of the signal void due to turbulence within the left atrium can be calculated based on multiple, contiguous slices in cine gradient echo. These parameters are directly related to the severity of the insufficiency. The size of signal void near the ventricular aspect of the valve can be used for the estimation of mitral regurgitation (Figure 4.9).

4.6   Pulmonary Regurgitation

Volume quantitation of pulmonary insufficiency by CMR can be accomplished by any of the previously described methods used for aortic insufficiency[17]. Regurgitant volume and regurgitant fraction calculation is carried out in the main pulmonary artery. The area below the diastolic curve of pulmonary flow corresponds to the pulmonary regurgitant flow. The regurgitant fraction is obtained from the division between the diastolic regurgitant volume and the ejection volume in systole (see Figure 8.22 in Chapter 8).

Pulmonary regurgitation is common in asymptomatic adults with repaired Tetralogy of Fallot. Severity of pulmonary regurgitation and its effects on right ventricular dimensions can accurately be assessed by CMR[18].

4.7   Pulmonary Hypertension

CMR allows access to many aspects of the function and anatomy of the right cardiac chambers that reflect the consequences of pulmonary hypertension. Dilatation of the vena cava, right chambers and of the pulmonary arteries are findings related to pulmonary hypertension that are easily demonstrated with CMR. In these patients, anomalies in the pulsatile flow of the pulmonary arteries with patterns of flow with inversion at the end of systole and in diastole are found, as well as an early systolic velocity peak[19]. Pulmonary hypertension is calculated using methods similar to those used in Doppler echocardiography: the tricuspid regurgitation velocity is calculated in order to estimate the systolic gradient between the right ventricle and atrium and, when the estimated pressure in the right atrium is added to this gradient, systolic pulmonary pressure can be derived, as long as pulmonary stenosis is not present.

4.8   Valvular Stenosis

a. Quantitation with cine velocity mapping

Valvular stenosis can be quantified by calculating the flow velocity, to which the simplified equation of Bernouilli is applied[20, 21], as is done in the Doppler technique. The spatial and temporal profile of blood velocity can be

FIGURE 4.6

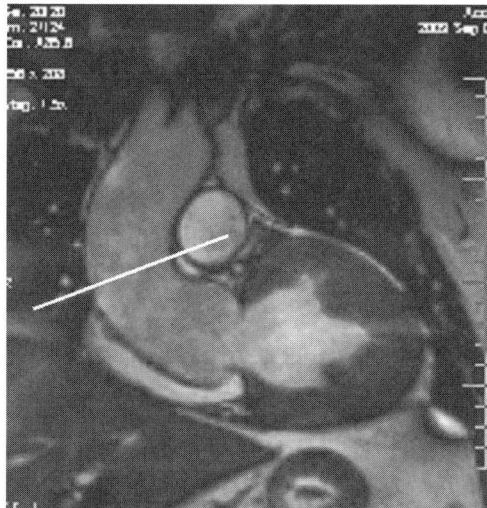

FIGURE 4.8

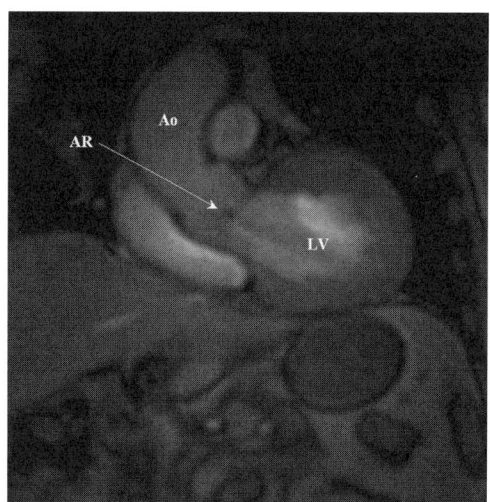

FIGURE 4.7

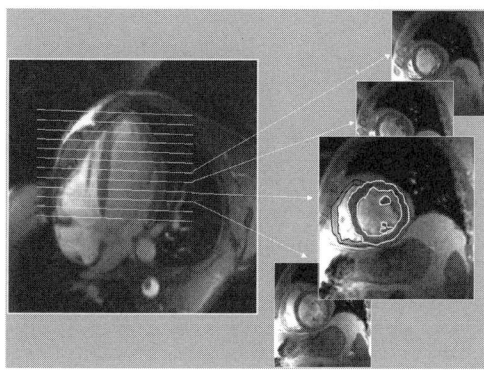

FIGURE 4.9

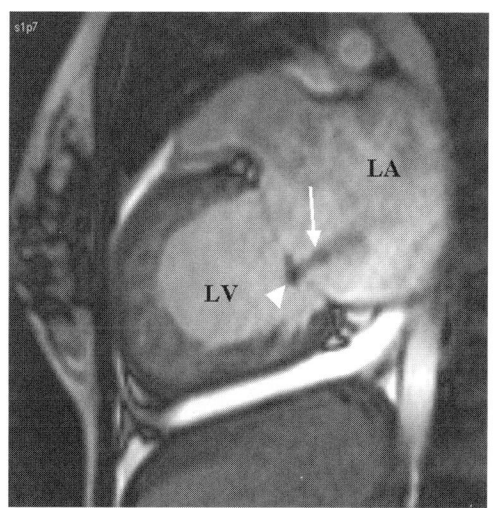

F. 4.6.   Coronal plane showing the orientation (line) of the phase-contrast study of flow in the ascending aorta.

F. 4.7.   Simpson method. Cine gradient echo images in 4 chambers view (left) and multiple parallel slices (right) in a sort axis view for segmentation of endocardial and epicardial edges in diastole and systole of both ventricles. Volumes are calculated by the sum of the areas estimated in every parallel slice multiply by the sum of its thickness and slap.

F. 4.8.   Aortic regurgitation. Diastolic frame of a cine gradient echo sequence in a plane perpendicular to the aortic valve plane. The signal void (AR) in the aortic side of the valve is produced by the acceleration of flow proximal to the valve defect. Ao: ascending aorta and LV: left ventricle.

F. 4.9.   Systolic frame from a cine MR sequence showing a signal of turbulent flow due to mitral regurgitation (arrow); note the signal void at the ventricular aspect of the valve plane (arrowhead). LA: left atrium; LV: left ventricle.

recorded in images obtained on planes including the stenotic flow direction previously identified with cine gradient-echo sequences. The behavior of the stenotic jet can be registered in cine, which provides information similar to color Doppler, but with significant differences. CMR maps can record velocities with practically no limits for the precise study of pathological hemodynamic gradients. Also, the possibility of analyzing the velocity in any spatial plane permits flow with any direction to be registered (Figures 4.3 and 4.4). The measurements of pressure gradients, velocity-time integral, and the valve dimension correlate well with the accepted standard of Doppler ultrasound[22].

b. Cine gradient echo

In normal subjects, a bright white signal is registered during valvular opening, generated by physiological laminar flow. During valvular opening, and occasionaly during its closure, transient turbulent signals that have no pathological significance may be recorded. Flow turbulence originated by valvular stenosis during opening is manifested as an area of signal void (Figures 4.3 and 4.4), represented in black in the cine gradient-echo images. The spatial and temporal magnitude of the area of turbulence registered in the cine image is related to the severity of the stenosis. The irregularities or anfractuosity of the calcified valvular leaflets contribute to the formation of turbulence and, on occasion, can magnify the signal void area in the cine image, with the result that the severity of the stenosis can be overestimated.

4.9 Prosthetic valves

Although there is occasionally concern in submitting patients with cardiac valve prosthesis to an CMR evaluation, the examination is in fact not contraindicated (except in the case of some old prostheses). Instead, the technique can even be useful in the evaluation of the function of the prosthesis.

There are in vitro studies validating the measurements of transprosthetic flow velocity registered with[23]. CMR evaluation of the dysfunction of the valvular prosthesis has an

excellent correlation with transesophageal echocardiography (TEE)[24]. The intra- or paraprosthetic origin of regurgitation with respect to differentiating physiological insufficiency (Figure 4.10) from prosthetic dysfunction can be evaluated with cine gradient-echo images (Cine Loop 4.04 on CD). The evaluation of the severity of the regurgitation jets according to the criteria of area or depth of turbulence also has a good correlation with TEE. Although TEE is still the technique of choice for the study of these patients, CMR represents a valid alternative for patients who refuse to undergo transesophageal exploration or when diagnostic limitations occur.

Transprosthetic gradient during valvular opening can be known by means of velocity maps and, also, quantitative methods pre-

FIGURE 4.10

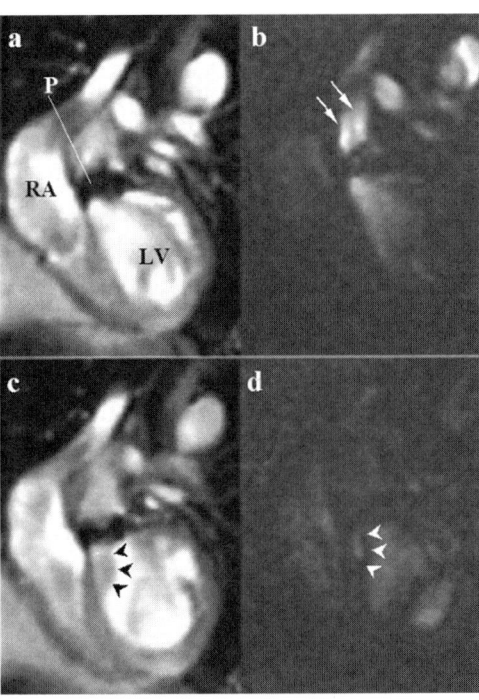

F. 4.10. Mechanical aortic prosthesis. Magnitude frames of a cine phase contrast sequence in a plane aligned with the prosthetic jet direction, in systole (a) and diastole (c). In diastole a physiological regurgitant jet is seen showing a small area of turbulence (arrowheads). Systolic (b) and diastolic (d) frames of velocity maps with velocity encoded in the same direction than the jets; two normal systolic jets (arrows) and one diastolic jet (arrowheads) of the prosthesis can be analyzed in phase contrast images. LV: left ventricle and RA: right atrium.

viously described for the calculation of regurgitation in native valves can also be employed in the case of valvular leaks.

References

1. Didier D. Assessment of valve disease: qualitative and quantitative. Magn Reson Imaging Clin N Am. 2003 Feb;11(1):115–34.

2. Friedrich MG, Schulz-Menger J, Poetsch T, et al. Quantification of valvular aortic stenosis by magnetic resonance imaging. Am Heart J. 2002; 144: 329–334.

3. Kupfahl C, Honold M, Meinhardt G, et al. Evaluation of aortic stenosis by cardiovascular magnetic resonance imaging: comparison with established routine clinical techniques. Heart. 2004; 90: 893–901.

4. Ichikawa Y, Sakuma H, Kitagawa K, et al. Evaluation of left ventricular volumes and ejection fraction using fast steady-state cine MR imaging: comparison with left ventricular angiography. J Cardiovasc Magn Reson. 2003; 5: 333–42.

5. Jiménez-Borreguero LJ, Kilner PJ, Firmin DN. Precision of magnetic resonance velocity mapping to calculate flow: an in vitro study. J Cardiovasc Magn Reson 1998; 1: 85.

6. Alfakih K, Plein S, Thiele H, Jones T, Ridgway JP, Sivananthan MU. Normal human left and right ventricular dimensions for CMR as assessed by turbo gradient echo and steady-state free precession imaging sequences. J Magn Reson Imaging. 2003; 17: 323–329.

7. John AS, Dill T, Brandt RR, et al. Magnetic resonance to assess the aortic valve area in aortic stenosis: how does it compare to current diagnostic standards?. J Am Coll Cardiol. 2003; 42: 519–526.

8. Caduff JH, Hernandez RJ, Ludomirsky A. MR visualization of aortic vegetations. J Comput Assist Tomogr. 1996;20:613–15.

9. Akins EW, Limacher M, Slone RM, Hill JA. Evaluation of an aortic annular pseudoaneurysm by MRI: comparison with echocardiography, angiography and surgery. Cardiovasc Intervent Radiol 1987;10:188–93.

10. Underwood SR, Klipstein RH, Firmin DN, et al. Magnetic resonance assessment of aortic and mitral regurgitation. Be Heart J 1986;56:455–62.

11. Sechtem U, Pflugfelder PW, Cassidy MM, et al. Mitral or aortic regurgitation: Quantification of regurgitant volumes with cine MR imaging. Radiology 1988;167:425–30.

12. Higgins CB, Wagner S, Kondo C, Suzuki J, Caputo GR. Evaluation of valvular heart disease with cine gradient echo magnetic resonance imaging. Circulation. 1991; 84(3 Suppl): I198–207.

13. Yoshida K, Yoshikawa J, Hozmi T, et al. Assessment of aortic regurgitation by the acceleration flow signal void proximal to the leak orifice in cinemagnetic resonance imaging. Circulation 1991;83:1951–55.

14. Jimenez-Borreguero LJ, Kilner PJ, Underwood SR, Firmin DN. Flow quantification with magnetic resonance using the isovelocity area method close to an orifice: an in vitro study. J Cardiovasc Magn Reson 1998;1:85.

15. Fujita N, Chazouilleres AF, Hartiala JJ, et al. Quantification of mitral regurgitation by velocity-encoded cine nuclear magnetic resonance imaging. J Am Coll Cardiol 1994;23:951–8.

16. Mohiaddin RH, Wann SL, Underwood R, Firmin DN, Rees S, Longmore DB. Vena caval flow: assessment with cine MR velocity mapping. Radiology. 1990; 177: 537–41.

17. Rebergen SA, Chin JG, Ottenkamp J, van der Wall EE, de Roos A. Pulmonary regurgitation in the late postoperative follow-up of tetralogy of Fallot. Volumetric quantitation by nuclear magnetic resonance velocity mapping. Circulation. 1993;88:2257–66.

18. Li W, Davlouros PA, Kilner PJ, et al. Doppler-echocardiographic assessment of pulmonary regurgitation in adults with repaired tetralogy of Fallot: comparison with cardiovascular magnetic resonance imaging. Am Heart J. 2004; 147: 165–72.

19. Kondo C, Caputo GR, Masui T, et al. Pulmonary hypertension: Pulmonary flow quantification and flow profile analisys with velocity-encoded cine MR imaging. Radiology 1992;183:751.

20. Kilner PJ, Manzara CC, Mohiaddin RH, et al. Magnetic resonance jet velocity mapping in

mitral and aortic valve stenosis. Circulation. 1993; 87: 1239–48.

21. Kilner PJ, Firmin DN, Rees RS, et al. Valve and great vessel stenosis: assessment with MR jet velocity mapping. Radiology. 1991; 178: 229–35.

22. Caruthers SD, Lin SJ, Brown P, et al. Practical value of cardiac magnetic resonance imaging for clinical quantification of aortic valve stenosis: comparison with echocardiography. Circulation. 2003; 108: 2236–43.

23. Walker PG, Pedersen EM, Oyre S, et al. Magnetic resonance velocity imaging: a new method for prosthetic heart valve study. J Heart Valve Dis. 1995; 4: 296–307.

24. Deutsch HJ, Bachmann R, Sechtem U, et al. Regurgitant flow in cardiac valve prostheses: diagnostic value of gradient echo nuclear magnetic resonance imaging in reference to transesophageal two-dimensional color Doppler echocardiography. J Am Coll Cardiol. 1992;19:1500–7.

Cardiovascular Magnetic Resonance of Ischemic Heart Disease

5

SANDRA PUJADAS
FRANCESC CARRERAS

5.1 Introduction

Cardiovascular magnetic resonance (CMR) offers a comprehensive morphological and functional evaluation of the heart[1] and some insight into the study of coronary circulation[2]. During the last 5 years, contrast-CMR has become an important tool in the assessment of patients with ischemic heart disease, providing information about function, perfusion and viability in a single study.

The tomographic and multiplanar imaging capabilities and the ability to perform cine-MR sequences in any spatial plane permits reliable and reproducible measurements of left ventricular volumes and mass without any geometrical hypothesis, as well as the determination of systolic wall thickening and regional wall motion abnormalities[3]. This requires the application of Simpson's rule by adding the myocardial volume directly calculated from each contiguous transversal section covering the whole left ventricle, as explained in chapter 2. An accurate and reproducible calculation of left ventricular mass and volume in patients who have suffered a myocardial infarction may be of great interest in the longitudinal follow-up studies of myocardial remodeling in relation to therapeutic intervention[4].

Contrast-CMR with delayed-enhancement studies allow the identification, location and quantification of myocardial necrosis, whereas dynamic studies to assess cardiac function and perfusion are possible under pharmacologic stress conditions[5]. On the other hand, image resolution is superior to echocardiography and it does not have its limitations, mainly due to the physical properties of diagnostic ultrasound.

5.2 Study of Ventricular Function

CMR has proven to be an effective, accurate and reproducible technique to determine the measurements and functional parameters of both ventricles[6–9]. For the assessment of wall motion several frames (usually between 16 to 30 are sufficient) are acquired at the same anatomical level during different phases of the cardiac cycle and displayed in a continuous loop format (cine-MR). New gradient-echo techniques such as steady-state free precession (SSFP) sequences have shortened significantly the acquisition time (by a factor of 2 to 3) at similar temporal and spatial resolutions, providing high contrast between intracavitary blood and the endocardium without the use of contrast agents, and allowing accurate delineation of the endo- and epicardium[10, 11] (Figure 5.1 and Cine Loop 5.1 on CD).

a. Global ventricular function

The most common and accurate[12] approach for calculation of global ejection fraction (EF) is the one based on the Simpson rule, which states that volume of an object can be estimated by taking the sum of the cross-sectional areas in each section and multiplying it by the section thickness. Sections are currently obtained in the short-axis view as it provides slices almost perpendicular to the myocardial walls for the largest part of the left ventricle (LV), except in the apex. Myocardial boundaries are, thus, better depicted and partial volume effects are significantly reduced.

For an accurate measurement of ventricular volume it is essential that the stack of short-axis slices covers the ventricle entirely from apex to base (Figure 5.2). A section thickness between 6 and 10 mm is used, and the gap between slices varies from no gap (consecutive slices) to 4 mm. Currently, a stack covering the whole ventricle can be achieved within just a few breath-holds (average of 5; less than 20 sec duration each). Latest technology innovations such as parallel imaging techniques (SENSE, ASSET, IPAT) and new rapid sequences such as SSFP (balanced-FFE, trueFISP, FIESTA), have considerably shortened time of cine-MR acquisition[10, 13, 14]. The method is highly reproducible due to the high resolution of the MR images[8]. CMR has also proven to be a first-choice technique to measure the volume and mass of the right ventricle (RV)[15, 16] which, due to its anatomical irregularities, requires the use of the Simpson's rule.

b. Regional ventricular function

An accurate assessment of regional myocardial function can be obtained by contour tracings of the endo- and epicardium on a cine-MR sequence, performed by means of dedicated software (Figure 5.3 and Cine Loop 5.2 on CD).

However, in practice, a reliable estimation of segmental wall motion can be performed visually on the series of short-axis cine sequences of the left ventricle.

Both necrosis and myocardial ischemia result in segmental wall motion abnormalities. Myocardial akynesia with segmental thinning of the myocardial wall is a fair sign of scar due to a chronic myocardial infarction[17]. However, chronic (hibernation or stunning) or acute myocardial ischemia, as well as a non-transmural myocardial infarction, may also present with segmental dysfunction, the simple measure of wall thickness or thickening not allowing an accurate distinction between viable and non-viable myocardial tissue.

Perfusion and delayed contrast-enhanced, as well as dobutamine-stress cine-MR studies are additional techniques that may be performed for an accurate assessment of myocardial function, including viability, either in chronic[18, 19] or in acute coronary syndromes[20].

c. Myocardial tagging

A unique feature of CMR is that it allows the myocardium to be magnetically labelled with a rectangular or radial grid acting as a marker of muscle deformation during contraction[21, 22] (Figure 5.4 and Cine Loop 5.3 and 5.4 on CD). This grid consists on a series of lines of presaturation that precede the acquisition of a cine sequence and persist for a brief period time along the cardiac cycle. From the changes in the shape of this grid, rotational and translational motion of the heart can be studied. The harmonic phase (HARP) method is a processing technique that permits rapid analysis of tagged cardiac magnetic resonance image sequences[23]. However, software for the quantitative analysis of the parameters derived from the tagged images is restricted to the research field, as it is not available in the commercial MRI workstations. Nevertheless, customized software is being developed by research teams interested in tagging research, in order to obtain quantitative information able for clinical practice applications. Tagging has been reported to be a unique tool for the non-invasive measurement of strain changes throughout the left ventricle during ischemia[24], the study of diastolic function[25] and, in particular, for the

FIGURE 5.1

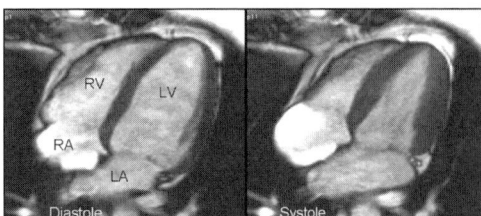

FIGURE 5.2

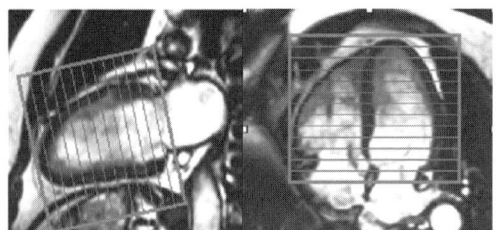

FIGURE 5.3

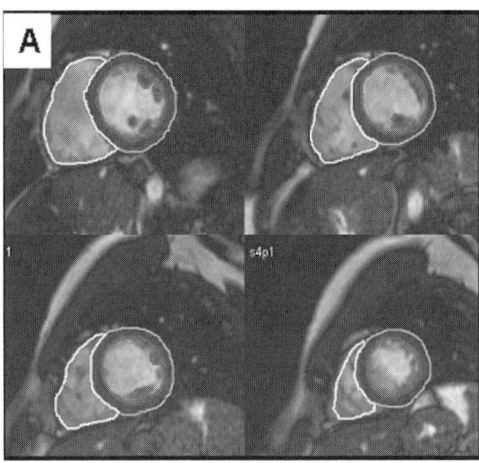

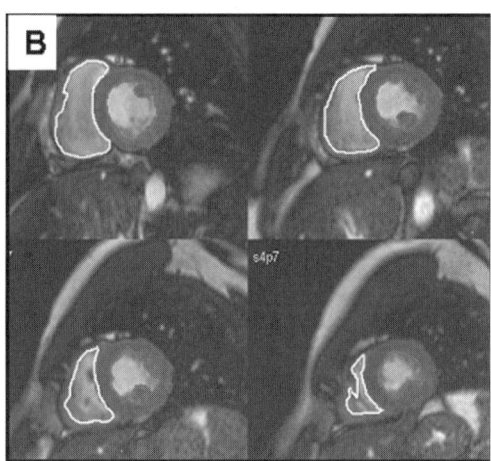

FIGURE 5.4

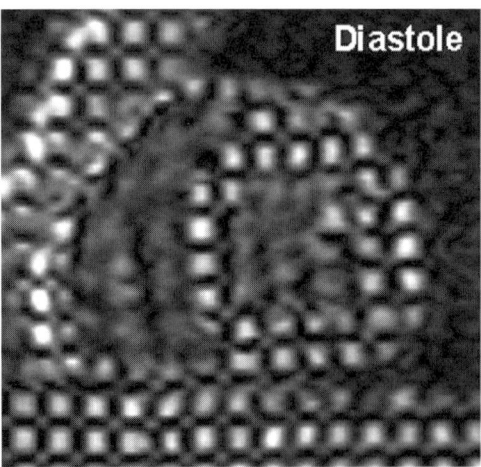

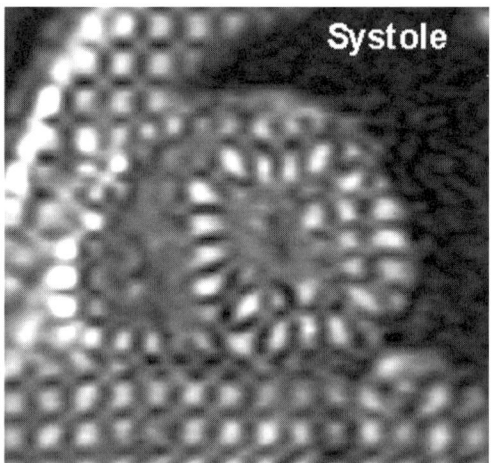

F. 5.1. Cine-MR of a ventricular horizontal long axis view (4 chamber) obtained with a SSFP sequence showing the excellent contrast between myocardium and blood.
LA: left atrium; LV: left ventricle; RA: right atrium; RV: right ventricle.

F. 5.2. Double oblique plane oriented along LV short-axis is prescribed using both long-axis images, vertical (2 chamber view) (on the left) and horizontal (4 chamber view) (on the right).

F. 5.3. Contours of the LV endo- and epicardium, as well as RV endocardium, might be traced through all diastolic (A) and systolic (B) cine-MR images using a dedicated software.

F. 5.4. Tagging images in a mid-ventricular short-axis section. A more accurate assessment of LV myocardial function may be obtained by analysing changes of tagged lines throught the systole.

better understanding of cardiac mechanics in normal[26] and pathological conditions[27].

5.3 Assessment of myocardial ischemia by stress CMR

On the basis of the "ischemic cascade"[28], we can approach the detection of myocardial ischemia by studying either myocardial perfusion or left ventricular contractility under pharmacological stress. There are two different types of pharmacological stress agents: vasodilators such as adenosine or dipyridamole, and beta agonists such as dobutamine. Vasodilators produce ischemia by means of a "steal" phenomenon in those territories with a reduced coronary flow reserve due to a severe coronary stenosis. On the other hand, dobutamine increases contractility and oxygen consumption, with a similar effect to that of exercise. In practice, vasodilators are used in perfusion studies, and dobutamine in the analysis of myocardial function under stress. The standard dose protocol for the intravenous administration of these agents and contraindications for their use are shown in Table 5.1.

Dobutamine stress studies are also useful to assess viability. The demonstration of the presence of myocardial contractile reserve by inducing an increase in systolic wall thickening by dobutamine is a highly accurate technique in comparison to F-18-FDG-uptake by PET for the identification of viable myocardium and prediction of functional recovery after successful revascularization[29]. Although myocardial wall thickness <5.5 mm excludes myocardial viability, a preserved end-diastolic wall thickness alone does not imply recovery of regional function. Dobutamine CMR may be helpful in these cases to increase the accuracy in the detection of myocardial viability[30, 31].

a. Myocardial perfusion by contrast first-pass CMR study

Contrast-enhanced CMR with gadolinium-DTPA has been demonstrated to be a feasible method for studying myocardial perfusion during the first pass of the agent through the myocardium (Figure 5.5 and cine Loop 5.5 on CD). Its clinical application is progressively increasing as an alternative to nuclear medicine for assessing microcirculation[32, 33], as well as for showing a better correlation with quantitative coronary angiography results than does stress enhancement SPECT[34]. Myocardial gadolinium concentration during first pass is determined primarily by myocardial blood flow[35] as 30–50% of the gadolinium chelate bolus enters myocardial interstitium on the first pass. In contrast with nuclear techniques, the myocardial concentration of gadolinium during first-pass does not depend on the integrity of myocardial cells[36].

Differences in myocardial perfusion can be detected by identifying the time changes of the myocardial signal intensity after contrast administration. The interpretation of the images can be done qualitatively by visual

Table 5.1 Doses and contraindications of pharmacological stress agents

	Doses	Contraindications
DOBUTAMINE	• Start: 10 µg/Kg/min • Maximal dose: 40 µg/kg/min • Increments: 10 µg/Kg/min every 3 minutes	Severe hypertension ($\geq$220/120 mmHg) Unstable angina pectoris Significant aortic stenosis Complex cardiac arrhythmias Hypertrophic obstructive cardiomyopathy Myocarditis, pericarditis, endocarditis
ADENOSINE	• 140 µg/Kg/min for 6 min	Unstable angina pectoris Severe hypertension Asthma or severe obstructive pulmonary disease
DIPYRIDAMOLE	• 0.56 µg/kg for 4 min	Atrioventricular block $\geq$IIa Carotid artery stenosis

assessment and classified as reversible (defect present only on stress imaging) (Figure 5.6 and Cine loop 5.6 and Cine loop 5.7 on CD) or fixed (present on stress and rest imaging). Semi-quantitative methods to assess myocardial perfusion reserve, by calculating the ratio of signal intensity curves obtained from the myocardial contrast enhancement before and after the administration of a vasodilator agent, have been also proposed (Figure 5.7). However, these methods are time-consuming and, at present, they are mainly restricted to the clinical research arena[37, 38].

To date, there is still debate on the most appropriate sequences to use for perfusion imaging, as the study of myocardial contrast during first-pass is the most demanding from a technical point of view. Different sequences have been proposed (see Ch 1) each group using the most suitable one according to their technical equipment and experience.

Practice of a CMR perfusion study

The detection of a regional myocardial perfusion defect with CMR first-pass gadolinium shows good diagnostic accuracy for the presence of significant coronary artery obstruction, provided that both rest and pharmacological stress studies are performed and perfusion is analyzed by semi-quantitative methods[39] and, also, with visual estimation of defects[40]. Rest acquisition is performed in multiple simultaneous sections prescribed in short axis views at different levels (basal, medium, apical). Optionally, we can also obtain long axis views. Gadolinium-based contrast is given as a compact intravenous bolus (better using a mechanical injector at 3 ml/s) at a dose of 0.02–0.05 mmol/kg. The injection is performed both at rest and under pharmacological stress, leaving a 10 minute interval between them to allow the contrast agent to be washed out from the myocardium after the first study. The basal and stress images are then compared for the assessment of perfusion defects.

b. Wall motion study by dobutamine-CMR

The reduction or absence of systolic myocardial thickening is the first functional marker of ischemia, which may be present even before electrocardiographic alterations[41]. Dobutamine-CMR is performed with an administration protocol similar to that normally used in echocardiographic studies[42]. However, dobutamine-CMR has demonstrated several advantages when compared to dobutamine-echocardiography. The excellent image quality allows an accurately assessment of the wall thickness and wall thickening due to a better delineation of the endocardial border than with echocardiography[43]. Therefore, reproducibility of the studies is highly superior than with echocardiography, and independent of the examiner.

In order to visualize all segments of the heart, a combination of several short-axis (typically basal, mid and apical) and horizontal and vertical long-axis views are acquired during the dobutamine infusion (Figure 5.8).

Safety is an important issue during the practice of dobutamine-CMR for the detection of myocardial ischemia, as potentially serious cardiovascular complications are expected in 0.25% of patients submitted to a maximal dobutamine stress test[44]. For this reason, patients must be closely monitored, and resuscitation equipment and trained personnel must be available.

Image analysis

For image interpretation a multiple cine loop display is required. Cine-loops of different stress levels are visualized and compared simultaneously allowing detection of new wall motion abnormalities. The left ventricle is analysed at 17 segments per stress level according to the standards suggested by the Cardiac Imaging Committee of the Council on Clinical Cardiology of the American Heart Association[45] (see Figure 2.16 in chapter 2). Segmental wall motion is classified qualitatively by visual estimation. Abnormal findings with increasing doses of dobutamine include reduction or lack of increase in systolic wall thickening in comparison with a previous level of stress. However, the clinical impact of CMR, in practice, for the diagnosis of coronary artery disease is still low. Further technical developments, including real time imaging and a reliable automated quantitative analysis of left ventricular function are required before dobutamine stress-CMR becomes a serious competition to stress-echocardiography on clinical grounds[46].

FIGURE 5.5

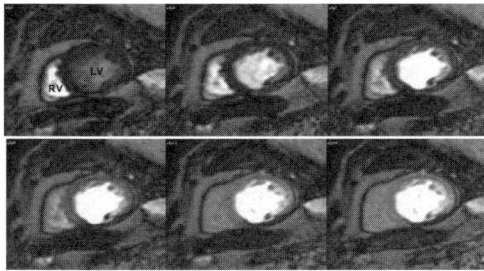

FIGURE 5.7

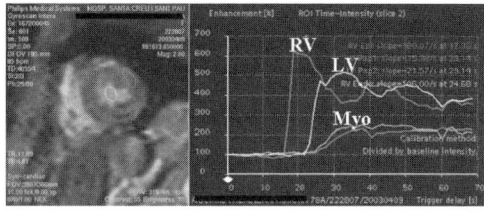

FIGURE 5.6

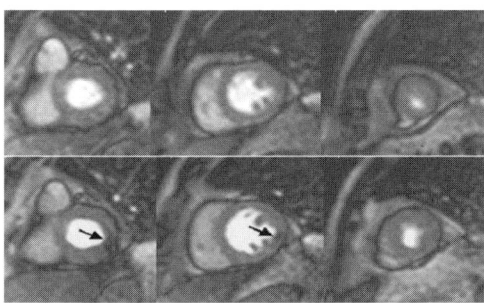

FIGURE 5.8

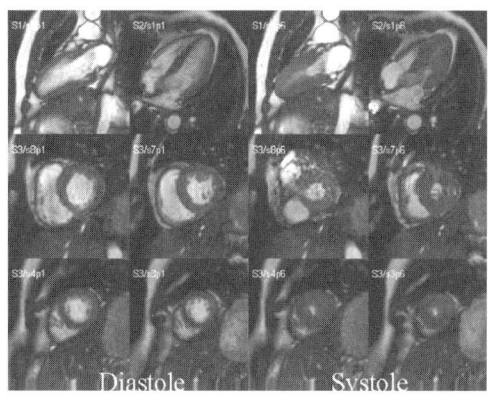

F. 5.5. Sequence of transit of contrast during a first-pass perfusion study. Initially, contrast agent enters cardiac chambers, resulting in a high signal intensity in the RV and, then, in the LV chamber, as opposed to the myocardium which remains dark (upper panel). Subsequently, the contrast agent will diffuse through the myocardium leading to a uniform increase in signal intensity throughout all the myocardial segments (lower panel).
LV, left ventricular chamber; RV, right ventricular chamber

F. 5.6. Perfusion study showing 3 short-axis sections (basal, mid and apical) acquired simultaneously during the first-pass of contrast agent. Upper panel, rest study (Cine Loop 5.6 on CD) shows no myocardial defects during gadolinium first-pass. Lower panel, stress study (Cine Loop 5.7 on CD) performed after adenosine perfusion shows a posterolateral hypoperfusion in the basal and mid myocardial segments (arrow).

F. 5.7. On the left a frame of a perfusion study is shown. Different regions of interest have been traced manually with a dedicated software in order to obtain time-signal intensity curves, as shown in the graph on the right. Observe the differences in timing and slopes of the curves from the right ventricular chamber (RV), the left ventricular chamber (LV), and the myocardium (Myo).

F. 5.8. Systolic and diastolic images of a Cine-MR dobutamine study. A combination of long axis (upper panel) and short-axis (mid and lower panel) views are displayed simultaneously in order to analyse segmental wall motion.

5.4 Acute and Chronic Myocardial Infarction

CMR can be used as a comprehensive examination in patients with infarction, assessing in the same study such different parameters as left ventricular shape, global and regional function, myocardial viability, and coronary artery patency[47].

Acute myocardial infarction can be directly identified on T2w SE images[48] due to the changes in myocardial relaxation times produced by the presence of myocardial edema (Figure 5.9). However, the frequently suboptimal quality of the image, degraded by the low signal-to-noise ratio of T2w sequences, does not permit a high diagnostic sensitivity with this method.

FIGURE 5.9

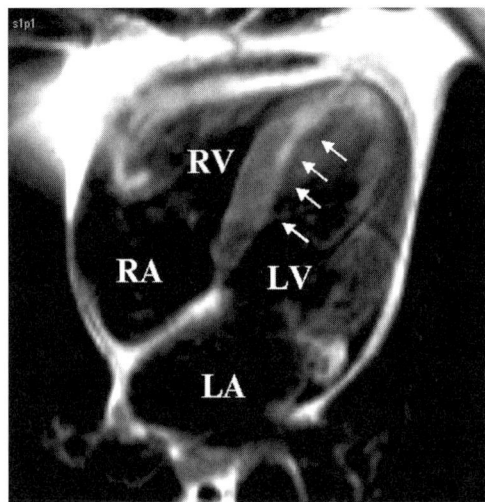

F. 5.9. Horizontal long-axis view T2w SE image of an acute septal myocardial infarction showing an area of higher signal intensity (arrows) corresponding to tissue edema. LA, left atrium; LV, left ventricle; RA, right atrium; RV right ventricle.

Excellent results in the identification and depiction of necrotic areas have been obtained by using quelated paramagnetic extracellular contrast agents, such as gadolinium-diethylenetriaminepenta-acetic acid (Gd-DTPA)[49]. Gadolinium-based contrast agent persists in the necrotic areas resulting in hyperenhancement, whereas it is rapidly removed ("washed-out") from viable myocardium, which shows lack of enhancement, provided the image acquisition is performed late in time (15 minutes after the constrast administration). The mechanisms at cellular level responsible for hyperenhancement are not fully understood. In acute infarction there is an increased volume of distribution of contrast due to interstitial edema and/or disruption of the myocyte membrane[35, 50, 51]. In chronic infarction, an explanation may be that interstitial space between collagen fibers in the scar tissue may be significantly greater than the interstitial space between myocytes in normal myocardium, this leading to a higher concentration of contrast agent in these areas compared to normal myocardium[52]. On the other hand, abnormal contrast molecule kinetics in infarcted/reperfused regions compared to normal have also been reported, showing a delayed contrast agent washout in these territories[53].

The development of a segmented inversion recovery sequence[54] significantly improved image quality and changed the potential of this technique to delineate necrotic areas. An inversion pulse is used with the inversion time (TI) set to null the signal from the normal myocardium, these areas appearing as dark. On the other hand, infarcted myocardium appears bright due to a shorter T1 associated with the contrast agent accumulation in these areas (Figure 5.10). Due to the excellent spatial resolution, as well as an important contrast between the hyperenhanced region (corresponding to myocardial infarction) and the null region (corresponding to normal myocardium), this technique has become the most accurate method for detecting and locating necrotic areas, as well as to determine its degree of transmurality (Figure 5.11)[49, 54, 55]. The optimal time window for imaging after contrast agent administration has been established between 6 and 25 minutes, as this is the time interval in which contrast between blood and enhanced myocardium is maximum[56]. Software packages available for clinical purposes allowing quantification of myocardial necrotic mass have been recently introduced (Figure 5.12), shortening the time analysis procedure.

The precise location[55] and quantitation[57] of the necrotic areas in the myocardium by means of delayed contrast-enhanced CMR has an important diagnostic and prognostic value[58, 59]. Since the introduction of this technique, CMR has dramatically increased its popularity and has emerged as a first-diagnostic tool on clinical grounds.

An important clinical contribution of delayed contrast-enhanced CMR is the detection of RV infarction[60]. It is well known that RV infarction is difficult to diagnose because it presents with transient ECG findings. Even echocardiography may miss the diagnosis in case of small infarctions with mild functional impairment. The excellent visualization of the RV free wall by CMR, as well as the high accuracy of the delayed contrast-enhanced method to detect necrotic tissue, has become the gold-standard for detection of RV infarction (Figure 5.13).

Also, recent studies have reported the applicability of CMR for the diagnostic assessment of acute coronary syndromes at the emergency department. Beek et al

FIGURE 5.10

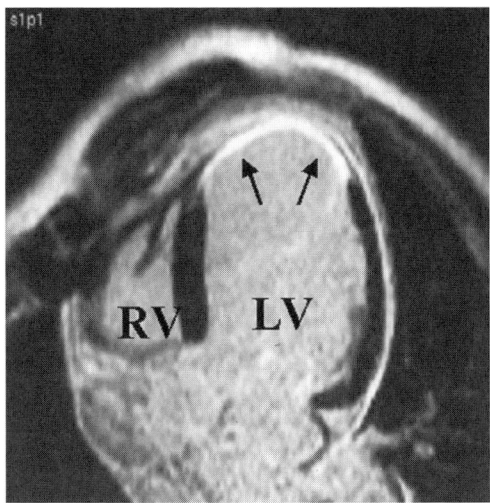

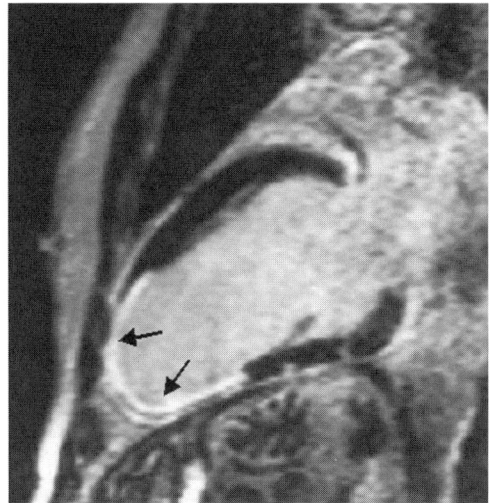

FIGURE 5.11

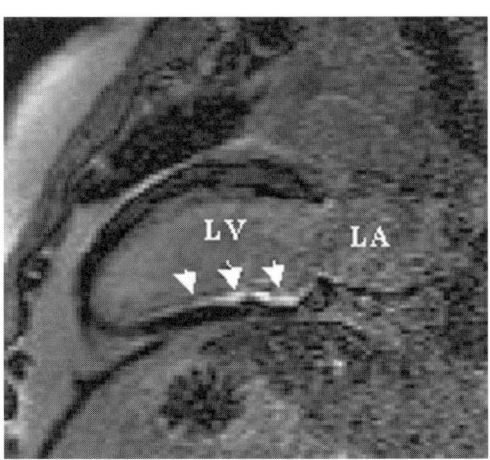

FIGURE 5.12

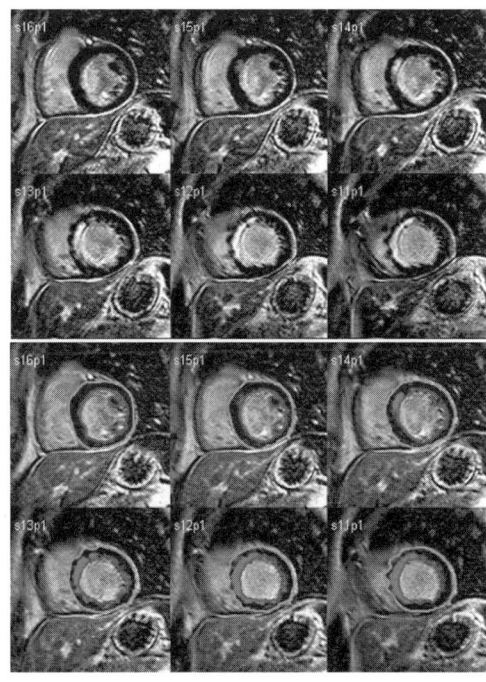

F. 5.10. Delayed contrast-enhanced images obtained with an inversion recovery sequence on a LV horizontal (left panel) and vertical (right panel) long-axis views showing an apical myocardial infarction. The infarcted region appears as "bright" (arrows), whereas normal myocardium shows no signal (dark) when using this particular sequence.
LV, left ventricle; RV, right ventricle

F. 5.11. Delayed contrast-enhanced image in a vertical long-axis section, showing a non-transmural infarction (arrows) of the inferior wall. The excellent spatial resolution of this type of sequence allows to accurately depict its extension within the myocardium.
LA, left atrium; LV, left ventricle

F. 5.12. Delayed contrast-enhanced short-axis images presenting an anterospetal infarction (bright myocardial area) (upper panel). By tracing endo- and epicardial contours, the myocardial area with a signal intensity above a threshold previously set is detected (lower panel) and, thus, necrotic myocardial mass can be calculated.

FIGURE 5.13

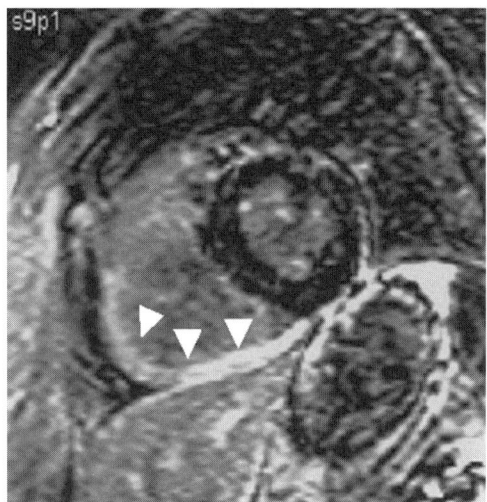

F. 5.13. Delayed contrast-enhanced image on a short axis view showing a bright myocardial signal in the RV free wall (arrow heads) corresponding to an isolated RV infarction.

showed[58] that CMR accurately identified a high proportion of patients with acute coronary syndrome, including those with enzyme-negative unstable angina.

5.5 Complications of Myocardial Infarction

Non-invasive imaging techniques have an important role for the detection of complications secondary to ischemic heart disease. A rationale use of echocardiography, CMR and, also, the recently introduced multidetector computed tomography, allow an optimal diagnostic assessment[61].

a. Ventricular aneurysm
SE and GRE techniques are useful for the detection of ventricular aneurysms and the delimitation of their extension (Figure 5.14 and Cine Loops 5.8 and 5.9 on CD), aiding in the surgical decision as well as in its technical planning. The ability of CMR to reproduce the same slice planes in serial studies improves the accuracy in the assessment of the anatomical changes after surgical correction (Figure 5.15)[62].

b. Subacute ventricular rupture and ventricular pseudoaneurysm
The noninvasive character of CMR and its high resolution to image paracardiac structures, as opposed to echocardiography, facilitates the assessment of left ventricular free-wall rupture after infarction (Figure 5.16), which may later evolve into the formation of a ventricular pseudoaneurysm (Figure 5.17 and Cine Loops 5.10 and 5.11 on CD). Delayed contrast-enhanced images may allow the distinction between the true necrotic tissue and the pseudoaneurysmal cavity (Figure 5.18).

c. Intraventricular thrombosis
Although intraventricular thrombus can be identified by T1w SE images (Figure 5.19), doubts may arise when flow artifacts are present in cases of aneurysmal ventricular dilatation and blood stagnation. The boundary between slow blood flow and the organized thrombus is somewhat difficult to establish on SE images[63]. In practice, GRE cine-MR sequences are helpful in distiguishing between a flow artifact and an organized thrombus[64] (Figure 5.20 and Cine Loop 5.12 on CD). Delayed contrast-enhancement studies are also able to depict mural thrombi in patients with myocardial infarction, usually located in left ventricular apex, presenting as dark well-defined structures surrounded by bright contrast-enhanced myocardium[65] (Figure 5.21). Tagging sequences may also be helpful in distinguishing between slow blood flow motion artifacts and thrombi, and it has been demonstrated to be especially useful when studying the thrombus content in aortic aneurysms, where flow stagnation is usual[66].

d. Mitral regurgitation
Although CMR is not the technique of choice for the diagnosis of mitral insufficiency, it is possible to identify its presence by means of cine sequences, as has been mentioned in chapter 4.

5.6 Assessment of myocardial viability

In patients with coronary artery disease (CAD) LV function is one of the major determinants

FIGURE 5.14

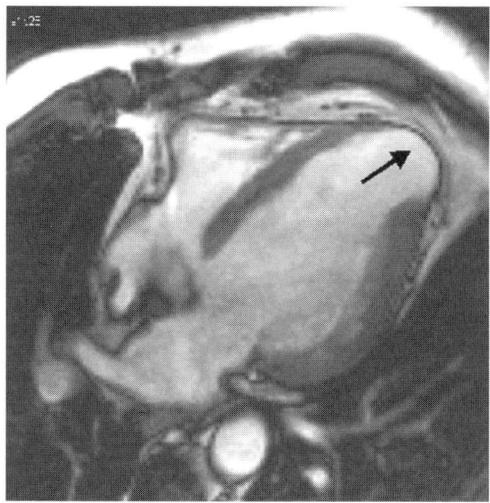 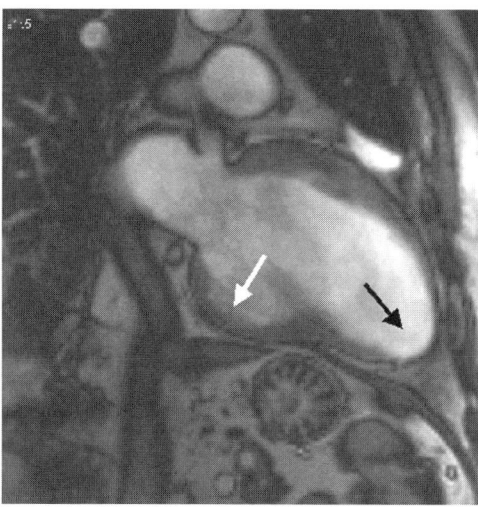

FIGURE 5.15

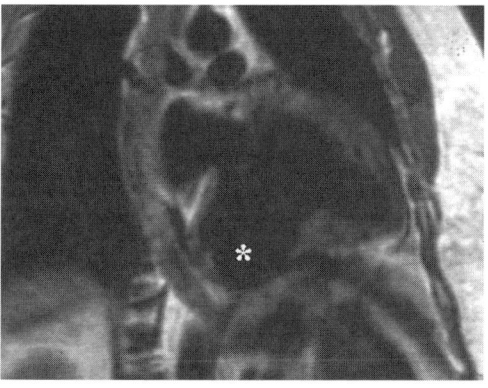 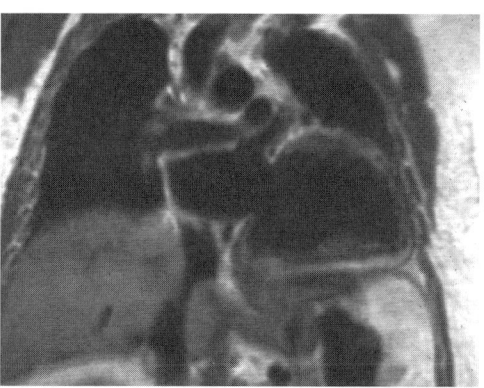

FIGURE 5.16

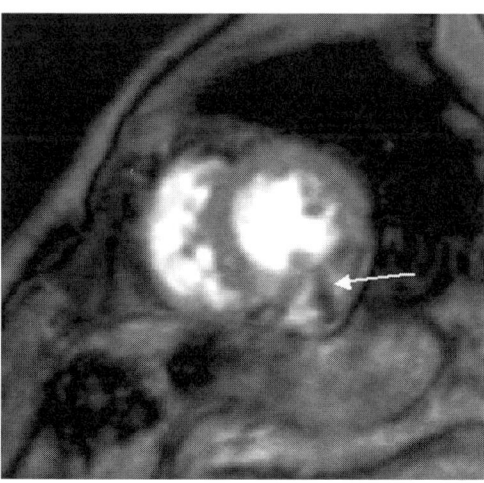 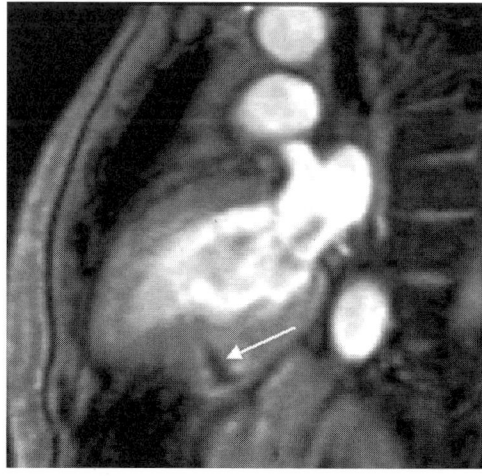

F. 5.14. On the left, a SSFP image obtained in a horizontal long-axis section showing an apical left ventricular aneurysm (black arrow). A vertical long-axis section obtained in the same patient is shown on the right panel. A second aneurysm located in the infero-basal wall is also visualized (white arrow).

F. 5.15. On the left panel, a vertical long-axis plane of the left ventricle showing a ventricular aneurysm of the infero-basal wall (asterisk). Note the indentation on the diaphragm caused by the aneurysm. On the right, an image from the same patient, with a same orientation, after surgical resection of the aneurysm.

F. 5.16. Left ventricular postinfarction rupture. Systolic images from a cine-MR GRE sequence obtained in a short-axis (left panel) and long-axis view (right panel) are presented, showing a flow signal of a turbulent jet (arrow) entering the psedoaneurysmal cavity from the true left ventricle.

FIGURE 5.17

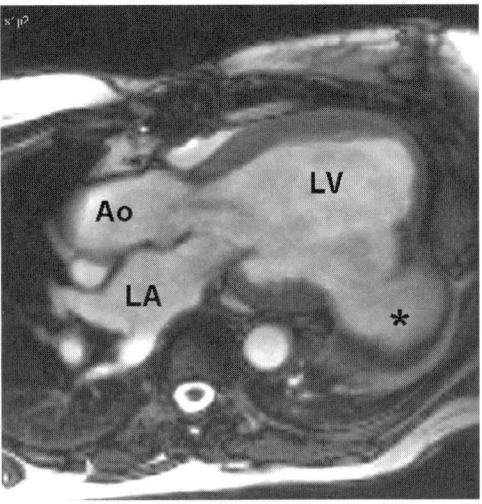

FIGURE 5.18

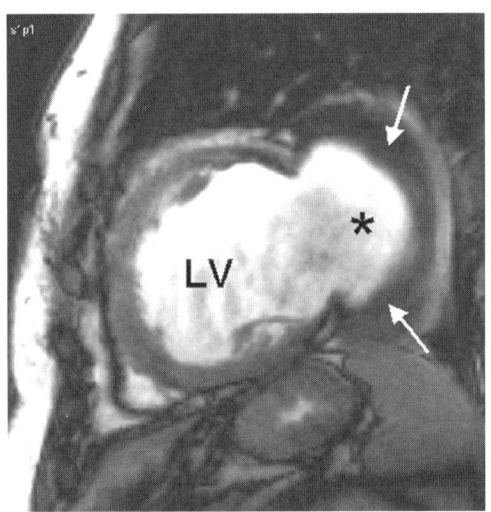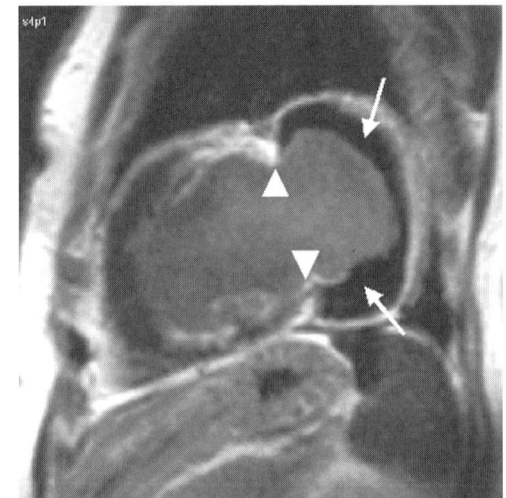

FIGURE 5.19

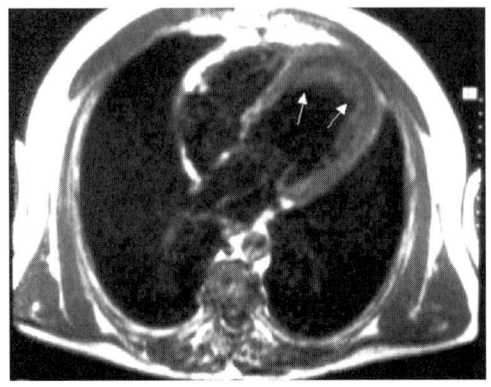

FIGURE 5.20

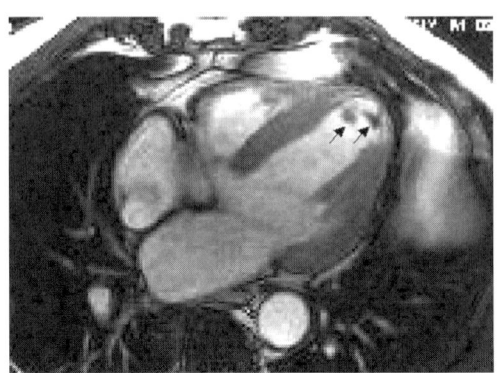

of long-term survival. Severe LV dysfunction results in poor prognosis[67–69]. However, myocardial dysfunction is not always an irreversible process. Reversible LV dysfunction in the presence of CAD include hibernation (impaired myocardial function at rest caused by chronic hypoperfusion) and stunned myocardium (contractile dysfunction that persists after severe or repetitive ischemia episodes despite of restoration of coronary blood flow). It is well established that LV dysfunction in the setting of CAD can improve following revascularization procedures[70–72]. Thus, determining viability in areas of severe regional dysfunction may be particularly important in patients with multivessel CAD in which coronary artery bypass graft surgery is contemplated. As mentioned above, delayed contrast-enhanced CMR can precisely identify necrotic areas[55, 73, 74]. Furthermore, it has been shown that the area at risk but not infarcted does not enhance[49, 75]. However, the most important feature regarding viability is the demonstration of a potential prediction of functional improvement after a revascularization procedure. Kim et al[76] showed that delayed contrast-enhanced CMR can identify reversible myocardial dysfunction before coronary revascularization. Regional dysfunction does not recover in regions with transmural hyperenhancement (Figures 5.22 and 5.23, and Cine Loops 5.13 and 5.14 on CD), whereas non-hyperenhanced dysfunctional myocardium improves after revascularization (Figures 5.24 and 5.25, and cine Loops 5.15 and 5.16 on CD). Moreover, transmurality extension of hyperenhancement is inversely related to improvement in wall thickening following revascularization (Figures 5.26 and 5.27, and cine Loops 5.17 and 5.18 on CD). However, although the absence of hyperenhancement in dysfunctional segments has demonstrated a high sensitivity for predicting contractile recovery[77], it has been reported that low-dose dobutamine-CMR is superior to delayed hyperenhancement as a predictor of recovery and does not depend on the transmurality of scar[78]. Although some controversy still remains on this topic[79], it has to be admitted that delayed contrast-enhanced CMR is safer, it requires less intense monitoring, it is easier to implement and faster to perform, and it also appears to be somewhat easier and faster to interpret than dobutamine-CMR.

No-reflow phenomenon can also be identified by delayed contrast-enhanced CMR as a dark region at the core of the infarct. Characteristically it is always surrounded by hyperenhanced tissue, as opposed to viable myocardium in which hyperenhancement is never seen in the epicardium (Figure 5.28). Microvascular obstruction or "no-reflow" has been shown to negatively influence left ventricular remodeling after myocardial infarction. The ability of delayed contrast-enhanced CMR to determine the extent of microvascular obstruction turns this technique into an important diagnostic and monitoring tool to assess the effectiveness of different therapeutic manoeuvres implemented in order to reduce the extension of the no-reflow area, as it has been described with the use of intra-aortic balloon counterpulsation[80].

In summary, CMR provides a unique tool to assess multiple interrelated clinical markers of viability in a single test. Its overall accuracy

F. 5.17.   Horizontal long-axis cine-MR image showing a posterolateral pseudoaneurysm (asterisk) of the left ventricle. High resolution CMR images allow a readily distinction between a true and a false aneurysm. Note in this case that the neck connecting the pseudoaneurysmal portion with the LV cavity is relatively narrow, and that the pseudoaneurysmal portion is contained by a very thin wall which is formed by adherent pericardium, these being characteristic findings of a pseudoaneurysm.
Ao: Aorta; LA: left atrium; LV: left ventricle

F. 5.18.   Short-axis view images from the same patient that in the previous figure, showing the ventricular pseudoaneurysm (asterisk) and a mural thrombus within its cavity (white arrows). Note the dark appearance of the thrombus on the cine-MR images (on the left) as opposed to the myocardium that shows an intermediate signal intensity. Delayed contrast-enhanced image (on the right) allows the distinction between necrotic myocardium, which shows a high signal intensity (arrow heads), and the pseudoaneurysm formed by pericardium, showing no delayed-enhancement. Thrombus do not show any signal in this type of sequence (appearing as dark), which may facilitate its identification.

F. 5.19.   T1w SE image on a long-axis plane showing an intraventricular laminar thrombus (white arrows) located into an apical aneurysm of the left ventricle.

F. 5.20.   SSFP cine-MR image showing apical thrombus (arrows).

FIGURE 5.21

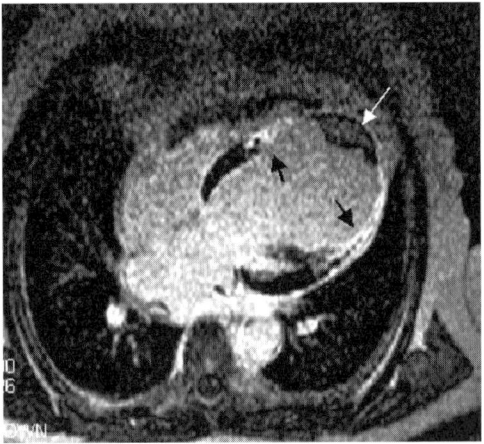

FIGURE 5.24

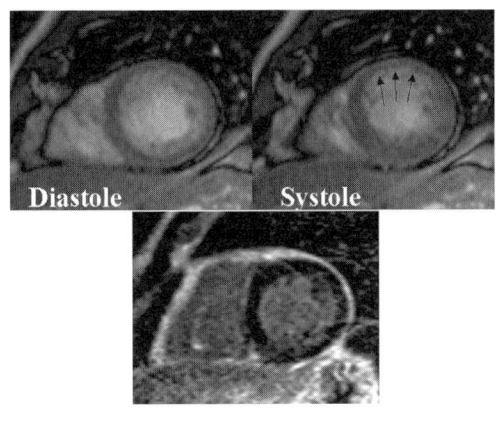

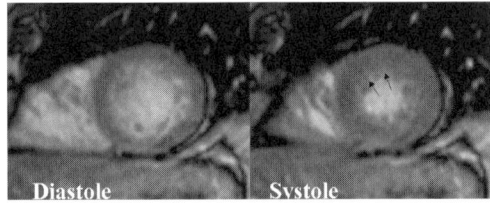

FIGURE 5.25

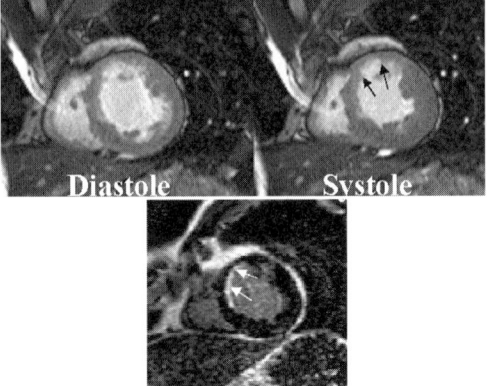

FIGURE 5.22

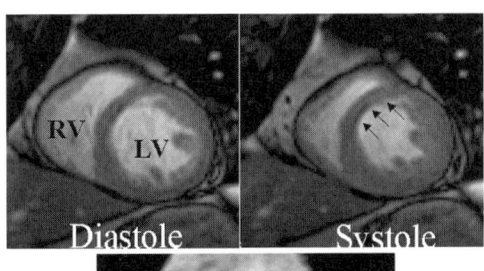

FIGURE 5.26

FIGURE 5.23

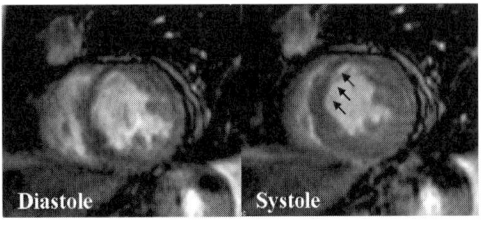

FIGURE 5.27

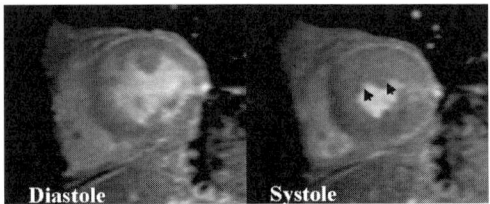

appears to be equivalent, and in several reports even superior, to the currently available techniques, including PET imaging[81].

Practice of a delayed contrast-enhanced study

A bolus of gadolinium-based contrast agent is administered intravenously by hand at 0.1–0.2 mmol/kg and images are acquired at 6–15 min later. Inversion-Recovery GE sequence with the inversion time (TI) set to null the signal in normal myocardium (typically 200–300 ms) is acquired. We will obtain the same views for the contrast-enhanced images as for the cine images so we can correlate motion-enhancement. It is important to note that no significant differences have been demonstrated when acquiring images 6 to 25 min after contrast administration[56]. However, the longer one waits after contrast administration, the longer TI delay should be set to obtain correct images. A thorough knowledge of the meaning of each pattern of myocardial enhancement is needed for an appropriate interpretation of results (Figure 5.29).

5.7 Imaging of Coronary Arteries

Despite the optimistic preliminary results published[82, 83], predicting a promising future for CMR as the first noninvasive technique able to visualize the coronary artery anatomy, technical problems remain preventing its use in clinical practice[84]. Recent improvements in MR hardware and software technology have provided extraordinary 3D images of the coronary tree (Figure 5.30)[85], however, time when coronary MR angiography (MRA) techniques will be a clinical routine is yet to come.

Coronary MRA involves an extraordinary challenge due to the small diameter of these vessels. Additionally, cardiac and respiratory motion have to be suppressed in order to obtain good image quality. In order to avoid cardiac motion, data should be acquired during a period in the cardiac cycle in which the coronary arteries are relatively quiescent: during isovolumic relaxation or in middiastole[86, 87]. Acquisition windows in the range of 70 − 100 ms are usually considered to be

F. 5.21.   Delayed contrast-enhanced long-axis image of a large left ventricular infarction showing an apical mural thrombus (white arrow). The necrotic area can be easily depicted due to its high signal intensity (bright) (black arrows).

F. 5.22.   Preoperative study of a patient with ischemic heart disease scheduled for coronary artery revascularization. On the upper panel, diastolic and systolic short-axis cine-MR images showing akynesia of the septal wall (Cine Loop 5.13 on CD). Lower panel, delayed contrast-enhanced image prescribed in the same section shows transmural delayed-enhancement in the septal wall (arrows) – showed as akynetic in the cine-MR images- indicating that this segment is not viable.
LV, left ventricle; RV, right ventricle

F. 5.23.   Cine-MR study of the same patient, performed 6 months after coronary artery revascularization surgery (Cine Loop 5.14 on CD). Note that septal wall persists akynetic confirming the absence of viability in this territory.

F. 5.24.   Cine-MR images (upper panel) from a patient with a severe LAD estenosis showing an anteroseptal diskynesia (Cine Loop 5.15 on CD). No delayed contrast-enhancement is observed (lower panel) indicating that this segment is potentially viable.

F. 5.25.   Cine-MR study of the same patient performed 4 weeks post-PTCA showed normal LV function by means of a complete recovery of the anteroseptal wall motion (Cine Loop 5.16 on CD).

F. 5.26.   Preoperative study of a patient with ischemic heart disease scheduled for coronary artery revascularization. Diastolic and systolic short-axis cine-MR images (upper panel) show an akynesia of the septal wall (Cine Loop 5.17 on CD). Delayed contrast-enhanced image prescribed in the same section (lower panel) shows non-transmural delayed-enhancement in the septal wall (arrows) –showed as akynetic in the cine-MR images- indicating that this segment is presumably viable.

F. 5.27.   Cine-MR study of the same patient performed 6 months after coronary artery revascularization surgery (Cine Loop 5.18 on CD) confirms septal wall viability by showing wall motion improvement of this segment post-revascularization.

FIGURE 5.28

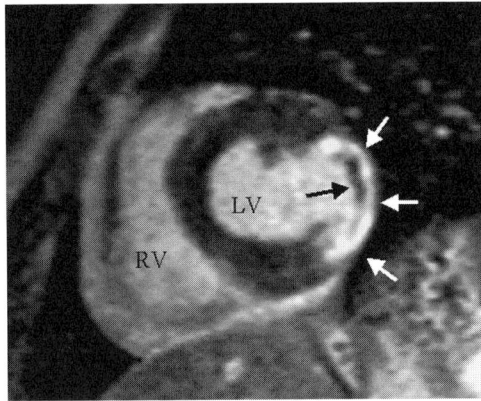

FIGURE 5.29

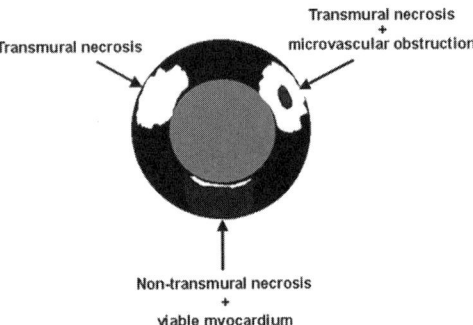

Transmural necrosis

Transmural necrosis
+
microvascular obstruction

Non-transmural necrosis
+
viable myocardium

FIGURE 5.30

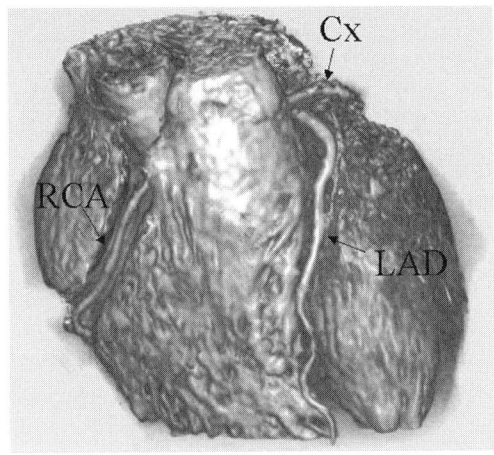

F. 5.28. Delayed contrast-enhanced image on a short-axis section showing lateral myocardial infarction as identified by means of a high signal intensity (white arrows). Note a dark core within the infarcted area (doughnut pattern) (black arrow), corresponding to an area of microvascular obstruction or "no-reflow".
LV, left ventricle; RV, right ventricle

F. 5.29. Different paterns of delayed contrast-enhancement distribution, which might be observed in patients with ischemic heart disease are shown.

F. 5.30. Three-dimensional rendered whole-heart coronary MRA (By courtesy of Oliver Weber, PhD, University of California, San Francisco).
Cx, circunflex coronary artery; LAD, left anterior coronary artery; RCA, right coronary artery

short enough for practical purposes. To avoid respiratory motion breath-holding approaches were initially used. However, the requirement of higher spatial resolution and improved 3D coverage prolonged acquisition times beyond the capabilities of breath-holding. Free-breathing approaches with navigator-based techniques serve to overcome the time constraint and the dependence on patient cooperation. Three-dimensional data acquisition enables data postprocessing by means of multiplanar reconstruction or maximum intensity projection to visualize the coronary arteries in different planes and orientations. Several approaches for 3D coronary imaging have been recently reported with encouraging results[85, 88–91]. Cartesian-turbo field echo is, however, the only sequence that has been evaluated in a relatively large multi-center study so far[92].

To date a maximum spatial resolution of 1 mm is achieved by coronary MRA as opposed to the 0.3 mm obtained by coronary angiography. Thus, though significant improvements in spatial and temporal resolution have been achieved, coronary MRA is not yet ready for clinical use for identification of focal coronary stenoses. Nevertheless, in experienced MR centers coronary MRA is accepted as the diagnostic method of choice in particular cases, such as in congenital anomalous coronary artery origin, or in the assessment and follow-up of coronary aneurysms.

In the recent years a competitive non-invasive technique such as multi-detector row computed tomography (MDCT) has emerged as the first-line technique for non-invasive coronary artery imaging[93, 94].

On the other hand, flow velocity assessment by means of MR phase velocity mapping sequences is an alternative method for the evaluation of vessel patency. Current described applications of this technique could be the detection of an open-artery after an acute

Table 5.2 Integrated -one-stop shop- study of ischemic heart disease using MRI

- Cardiovascular anatomic morphology (size of cavities, thickness of ventricular walls, ventricular mass, post-AMI remodeling, thrombus)- Global and regional ventricular contractility
- Myocardial perfusion studies with paramagnetic contrasts, at rest and under pharmalogical stress
- Morphologic assessment of the coronary tree and assessment of coronary artery bypass graft patency and function
- Myocardial metabolism study by MR spectroscopy

myocardial infarction[95], or the evaluation of the coronary artery bypass graft patency, whether they are saphenous vein grafts or internal mammary artery grafts[96, 97]. It should be kept in mind that the identification of a coronary vessel or a bypass graft depends on the presence of flowing blood in its lumen, since this is the target of MR techniques, producing the typical black blood flow signal in SE imaging or an intense bright blood flow signal in GRE imaging. Provided a good quality image, the lack of recognition of a bypass graft in its expected place would predict its occlusion.

In conclusion, CMR is a technique with an extraordinary potential for the study of ischemic heart disease, due to the broad spectrum of information it can provide and to its noninvasive nature. At present, CMR is undergoing a period of rapid technical development, a process that is favoured by the increasing number of cardiologists who are interested in its application[98]. Improvements in magnetic resonance hardware, software and imaging speed currently permit the assessment of LV function, ischemia and viability in one single study, which has made CMR to be known as a "one-stop-shop" technique[99, 100] (Table 5.2). Moreover, recent work in the molecular imaging field has demonstrated the feasibility of direct imaging of acute and subacute thrombosis using MR imaging together with a novel fibrin-binding gadolinium-labeled peptide[101]. Room is opened for the identification of the unstable plaque in acute and subacute coronary syndromes.

References

1. Budinger TF, Berson A, McVeigh ER, Pettigrew RI, Pohost GM, Watson JT, Wickline SA. Cardiac MR imaging: report of a working group sponsored by the National Heart, Lung, and Blood Institute. Radiology 1998;208(3):573–6.

2. van der Wall EE, Vliegen HW, de Roos A, Bruschke AV. Magnetic resonance imaging in coronary artery disease. Circulation 1995;92(9):2723–39.

3. Boxerman JL, Mosher TJ, McVeigh ER, Atalar E, Lima JA, Bluemke DA. Advanced MR imaging techniques for evaluation of the heart and great vessels. Radiographics 1998;18(3):543–64.

4. Foster RE, Johnson DB, Barilla F, Blackwell GG, Orr R, Roney M, Stanley AW, Jr., Pohost GM, Dell'Italia LJ. Changes in left ventricular mass and volumes in patients receiving angiotensin-converting enzyme inhibitor therapy for left ventricular dysfunction after Q-wave myocardial infarction. Am Heart J 1998;136(2):269–75.

5. de Roos A, Niezen RA, Lamb HJ, Dendale P, Reiber JH, van der Wall EE. MR of the heart under pharmacologic stress. Cardiol Clin 1998;16(2):247–65.

6. Semelka RC, Tomei E, Wagner S, Mayo J, Caputo G, O'Sullivan M, Parmley WW, Chatterjee K, Wolfe C, Higgins CB. Interstudy reproducibility of dimensional and functional measurements between cine magnetic resonance studies in the morphologically abnormal left ventricle. Am Heart J 1990;119(6):1367–73.

7. Semelka RC, Tomei E, Wagner S, Mayo J, Kondo C, Suzuki J, Caputo GR, Higgins CB. Normal left ventricular dimensions and function: interstudy reproducibility of measurements with cine MR imaging. Radiology 1990;174(3 Pt 1):763–8.

8. Pattynama PM, Lamb HJ, van der Velde EA, van der Wall EE, de Roos A. Left ventricular measurements with cine and spin-echo MR imaging: a study of reproducibility with variance component analysis. Radiology 1993;187(1):261–8.

9. Sakuma H, Fujita N, Foo TK, Caputo GR, Nelson SJ, Hartiala J, Shimakawa A, Higgins CB. Evaluation of left ventricular volume and mass with breath-hold cine MR imaging. Radiology 1993;188(2):377–80.

10. Barkhausen J, Ruehm SG, Goyen M, Buck T, Laub G, Debatin JF. MR evaluation of ventricular function: true fast imaging with steady- state precession versus fast low-angle shot cine MR imaging: feasibility study. Radiology 2001;219(1):264–9.

11. Lee VS, Resnick D, Bundy JM, Simonetti OP, Lee P, Weinreb JC. Cardiac function: MR evaluation in one breath hold with real-time true fast imaging with steady-state precession. Radiology 2002;222(3):835–42.

12. Dulce MC, Mostbeck GH, Friese KK, Caputo GR, Higgins CB. Quantification of the left ventricular volumes and function with cine MR imaging: comparison of geometric models with three-dimensional data. Radiology 1993;188(2):371–6.

13. Li W, Stern JS, Mai VM, Pierchala LN, Edelman RR, Prasad PV. MR assessment of left ventricular function: quantitative comparison of fast imaging employing steady-state acquisition (FIESTA) with fast gradient echo cine technique. J Magn Reson Imaging 2002;16(5):559–64.

14. Plein S, Bloomer TN, Ridgway JP, Jones TR, Bainbridge GJ, Sivananthan MU. Steady-state free precession magnetic resonance imaging of the heart: comparison with segmented k-space gradient-echo imaging. J Magn Reson Imaging 2001;14(3):230–6.

15. Pattynama PM, Lamb HJ, Van der Velde EA, Van der Geest RJ, Van der Wall EE, De Roos A. Reproducibility of MRI-derived measurements of right ventricular volumes and myocardial mass. Magn Reson Imaging 1995;13(1):53–63.

16. Grothues F, Moon JC, Bellenger NG, Smith GS, Klein HU, Pennell DJ. Interstudy reproducibility of right ventricular volumes, function, and mass with cardiovascular magnetic resonance. Am Heart J 2004;147(2):218–23.

17. Baer FM, Theissen P, Voth E, Schneider CA, Schicha H, Sechtem U. Morphologic correlate of pathologic Q waves as assessed by gradient-echo magnetic resonance imaging. Am J Cardiol 1994;74(5):430–4.

18. Baer FM, Theissen P, Schneider CA, Voth E, Sechtem U, Schicha H, Erdmann E. Dobutamine magnetic resonance imaging predicts contractile recovery of chronically dysfunctional myocardium after successful revascularization. J Am Coll Cardiol 1998;31(5):1040–8.

19. Baer FM, Erdmann E. Methods of assessment and clinical relevance of myocardial hibernation and stunning. Assessment of myocardial viability. Thorac Cardiovasc Surg 1998;46 Suppl 2:264–9.

20. Kwong RY, Schussheim AE, Rekhraj S, Aletras AH, Geller N, Davis J, Christian TF, Balaban RS, Arai AE. Detecting acute coronary syndrome in the emergency department with cardiac magnetic resonance imaging. Circulation 2003;107(4):531–7.

21. Zerhouni EA, Parish DM, Rogers WJ, Yang A, Shapiro EP. Human heart: tagging with MR imaging--a method for noninvasive assessment of myocardial motion. Radiology 1988;169(1):59–63.

22. Axel L, Dougherty L. Heart wall motion: improved method of spatial modulation of magnetization for MR imaging. Radiology 1989;172(2):349–50.

23. Osman NF, Kerwin WS, McVeigh ER, Prince JL. Cardiac motion tracking using CINE harmonic phase (HARP) magnetic resonance imaging. Magn Reson Med 1999;42(6):1048–60.

24. Moore CC, McVeigh ER, Zerhouni EA. Noninvasive measurement of three-dimensional myocardial deformation with tagged magnetic resonance imaging during graded local ischemia. J Cardiovasc Magn Reson 1999;1(3):207–22.

25. Nagel E, Stuber M, Burkhard B, Fischer SE, Scheidegger MB, Boesiger P, Hess OM. Cardiac rotation and relaxation in patients with aortic valve stenosis. Eur Heart J 2000;21(7):582–9.

26. Moore CC, McVeigh ER, Zerhouni EA. Quantitative tagged magnetic resonance imaging of the normal human left ventricle. Top Magn Reson Imaging 2000;11(6):359–71.

27. Kraitchman DL, Hillenbrand HB, Oznur I, Lima JA, McVeigh ER, Zerhouni EA, Bluemke DA. Noninvasive assessment of myocardial stunning from short-term coronary occlusion using tagged magnetic resonance imaging. J Cardiovasc Magn Reson 2000;2(2):123–36.

28. Nesto RW, Kowalchuk GJ. The ischemic cascade: temporal sequence of hemodynamic, electrocardiographic and symptomatic expressions of ischemia. Am J Cardiol 1987;59(7):23C–30C.

29. Schmidt M, Voth E, Schneider CA, Theissen P, Wagner R, Baer FM, Schicha H. F-18-FDG uptake is a reliable predictory of functional recovery of akinetic but viable infarct regions as defined by magnetic resonance imaging before and after revascularization. Magn Reson Imaging 2004;22(2):229–36.

30. Kaandorp TA, Bax JJ, Schuijf JD, Viergever EP, van Der Wall EE, de Roos A, Lamb HJ. Head-to-head comparison between contrast-enhanced magnetic resonance imaging and dobutamine magnetic resonance imaging in men with ischemic cardiomyopathy. Am J Cardiol 2004;93(12):1461–4.

31. Motoyasu M, Sakuma H, Ichikawa Y, Ishida N, Uemura S, Okinaka T, Isaka N, Takeda K, Nakano T. Prediction of regional functional recovery after acute myocardial infarction with low dose dobutamine stress cine MR imaging and contrast enhanced MR imaging. J Cardiovasc Magn Reson 2003;5(4):563–74.

32. Al-Saadi N, Nagel E, Gross M, Schnackenburg B, Paetsch I, Klein C, Fleck E. Improvement of myocardial perfusion reserve early after coronary intervention: assessment with cardiac magnetic resonance imaging. J Am Coll Cardiol 2000;36(5):1557–64.

33. Panting JR, Gatehouse PD, Yang GZ, Grothues F, Firmin DN, Collins P, Pennell DJ. Abnormal subendocardial perfusion in cardiac syndrome X detected by cardiovascular magnetic resonance imaging. N Engl J Med 2002;346(25):1948–53.

34. Ishida N, Sakuma H, Motoyasu M, Okinaka T, Isaka N, Nakano T, Takeda K. Noninfarcted myocardium: correlation between dynamic first-pass contrast-enhanced myocardial MR imaging and quantitative coronary angiography. Radiology 2003;229(1):209–16.

35. Diesbourg LD, Prato FS, Wisenberg G, Drost DJ, Marshall TP, Carroll SE, O'Neill B. Quantification of myocardial blood flow and extracellular volumes using a bolus injection of Gd-DTPA: kinetic modeling in canine ischemic disease. Magn Reson Med 1992;23(2):239–53.

36. Barkhausen J, Hunold P, Jochims M, Debatin JF. Imaging of myocardial perfusion with magnetic resonance. J Magn Reson Imaging 2004;19(6):750–7.

37. Doyle M, Fuisz A, Kortright E, Biederman RW, Walsh EG, Martin ET, Tauxe L, Rogers WJ, Merz CN, Pepine C, Sharaf B, Pohost GM. The impact of myocardial flow reserve on the detection of coronary artery disease by perfusion imaging methods: an NHLBI WISE study. J Cardiovasc Magn Reson 2003;5(3):475–85.

38. Jerosch-Herold M, Seethamraju RT, Swingen CM, Wilke NM, Stillman AE. Analysis of myocardial perfusion MRI. J Magn Reson Imaging 2004;19(6):758–70.

39. Schwitter J, Nanz D, Kneifel S, Bertschinger K, Buchi M, Knusel PR, Marincek B, Luscher TF, von Schulthess GK. Assessment of myocardial perfusion in coronary artery disease by magnetic resonance: a comparison with positron emission tomography and coronary angiography. Circulation 2001;103(18):2230–5.

40. Pons Llado G, Carreras F, Leta R, Pujadas S, Garcia Picart J. [Assessment of myocardial perfusion by cardiovascular magnetic resonance: comparison with coronary angiography]. Rev Esp Cardiol 2004;57(5):388–95.

41. Upton MT, Rerych SK, Newman GE, Port S, Cobb FR, Jones RH. Detecting abnormalities in left ventricular function during exercise before angina and ST-segment depression. Circulation 1980;62(2):341–9.

42. Baer FM, Voth E, Theissen P, Schicha H, Sechtem U. Gradient-echo magnetic resonance imaging during incremental dobutamine infusion for the localization of coronary artery stenoses. Eur Heart J 1994;15(2):218–25.

43. Nagel E, Lehmkuhl HB, Bocksch W, Klein C, Vogel U, Frantz E, Ellmer A, Dreysse S, Fleck E. Noninvasive diagnosis of ischemia-induced wall motion abnormalities with the use of high-dose dobutamine stress MRI: comparison with dobutamine stress echocardiography. Circulation 1999;99(6):763–70.

44. Wahl A, Paetsch I, Gollesch A, Roethemeyer S, Foell D, Gebker R, Langreck H, Klein C, Fleck E, Nagel E. Safety and feasibility of high-dose dobutamine-atropine stress cardiovascular magnetic resonance for diagnosis of myocardial ischaemia: experience in 1000 consecutive cases. Eur Heart J 2004;25(14):1230–6.

45. Cerqueira MD, Weissman NJ, Dilsizian V, Jacobs AK, Kaul S, Laskey WK, Pennell DJ,

Rumberger JA, Ryan T, Verani MS. Standardized myocardial segmentation and nomenclature for tomographic imaging of the heart: a statement for healthcare professionals from the Cardiac Imaging Committee of the Council on Clinical Cardiology of the American Heart Association. Circulation 2002;105(4):539–42.

46. Baer FM, Crnac J, Schmidt M, Jochims M, Theissen P, Schneider C, Schicha H, Erdmann E. Magnetic resonance pharmacological stress for detecting coronary disease. Comparison with echocardiography. Herz 2000;25(4):400–8.

47. Kramer CM, Rogers WJ, Geskin G, Power TP, Theobald TM, Hu YL, Reichek N. Usefulness of magnetic resonance imaging early after acute myocardial infarction. Am J Cardiol 1997;80(6):690–5.

48. Garcia-Dorado D, Oliveras J, Gili J, Sanz E, Perez-Villa F, Barrabes J, Carreras MJ, Solares J, Soler-Soler J. Analysis of myocardial oedema by magnetic resonance imaging early after coronary artery occlusion with or without reperfusion. Cardiovasc Res 1993;27(8):1462–9.

49. Kim RJ, Fieno DS, Parrish TB, Harris K, Chen EL, Simonetti O, Bundy J, Finn JP, Klocke FJ, Judd RM. Relationship of MRI delayed contrast enhancement to irreversible injury, infarct age, and contractile function. Circulation 1999;100(19):1992–2002.

50. Schwitter J, Saeed M, Wendland MF, Derugin N, Canet E, Brasch RC, Higgins CB. Influence of severity of myocardial injury on distribution of macromolecules: extravascular versus intravascular gadolinium-based magnetic resonance contrast agents. J Am Coll Cardiol 1997;30(4):1086–94.

51. Saeed M, Wendland MF, Masui T, Higgins CB. Reperfused myocardial infarctions on T1- and susceptibility-enhanced MRI: evidence for loss of compartmentalization of contrast media. Magn Reson Med 1994;31(1):31–9.

52. Kim RJ, Choi KM, Judd RM. Assessment of myocardial viability by contrast enhancement. In: Higgins CB, De Roos A, eds. Cardiovascular MRI and MRA. Philadelphia, PA: Lippincott Williams & Wilkins; 2002:209–37.

53. Kim RJ, Chen EL, Lima JA, Judd RM. Myocardial Gd-DTPA kinetics determine MRI contrast enhancement and reflect the extent and severity of myocardial injury after acute reperfused infarction. Circulation 1996;94(12):3318–26.

54. Simonetti OP, Kim RJ, Fieno DS, Hillenbrand HB, Wu E, Bundy JM, Finn JP, Judd RM. An improved MR imaging technique for the visualization of myocardial infarction. Radiology 2001;218(1):215–23.

55. Wu E, Judd RM, Vargas JD, Klocke FJ, Bonow RO, Kim RJ. Visualisation of presence, location, and transmural extent of healed Q-wave and non-Q-wave myocardial infarction. Lancet 2001;357(9249):21–8.

56. Grebe O, Paetsch I, Kestler HA, Herkommer B, Schnackenburg B, Hombach V, Fleck E, Nagel E. Optimal acquisition parameters for contrast enhanced magnetic resonance imaging after chronic myocardial infarction. J Cardiovasc Magn Reson 2003;5(4):575–87.

57. Ingkanisorn WP, Rhoads KL, Aletras AH, Kellman P, Arai AE. Gadolinium delayed enhancement cardiovascular magnetic resonance correlates with clinical measures of myocardial infarction. J Am Coll Cardiol 2004;43(12):2253–9.

58. Beek AM, Kuhl HP, Bondarenko O, Twisk JW, Hofman MB, van Dockum WG, Visser CA, van Rossum AC. Delayed contrast-enhanced magnetic resonance imaging for the prediction of regional functional improvement after acute myocardial infarction. J Am Coll Cardiol 2003;42(5):895–901.

59. Choi KM, Kim RJ, Gubernikoff G, Vargas JD, Parker M, Judd RM. Transmural extent of acute myocardial infarction predicts long-term improvement in contractile function. Circulation 2001;104(10):1101–7.

60. Finn AV, Antman EM. Images in clinical medicine. Isolated right ventricular infarction. N Engl J Med 2003;349(17):1636.

61. White RD. MR and CT assessment for ischemic cardiac disease. J Magn Reson Imaging 2004;19(6):659–75.

62. Setser RM, White RD, Sturm B, McCarthy PM, Starling RC, Young JB, Kasper J, Buda T, Obuchowski N, Lieber ML. Noninvasive assessment of cardiac mechanics and clinical outcome after partial left ventriculectomy. Ann Thorac Surg 2003;76(5):1576–85; discussion 85–6.

63. Chung JW, Park JH, Han JK, Kim HC, Han MC. Hypointense boundary layer between slow flow and mural thrombus on spin-echo MR. J Comput Assist Tomogr 1992;16(6):944–50.

64. Jungehulsing M, Sechtem U, Theissen P, Hilger HH, Schicha H. Left ventricular thrombi: evaluation with spin-echo and gradient-echo MR imaging. Radiology 1992;182(1):225–9.

65. Mollet NR, Dymarkowski S, Volders W, Wathiong J, Herbots L, Rademakers FE, Bogaert J. Visualization of ventricular thrombi with contrast-enhanced magnetic resonance imaging in patients with ischemic heart disease. Circulation 2002;106(23):2873–6.

66. Honda T, Hamada M, Matsumoto Y, Matsuoka H, Hiwada K. Diagnosis of Thrombus and Blood Flow in Aortic Aneurysm Using Tagging Cine Magnetic Resonance Imaging. International Journal of Angiology 1999;8(1):57–61.

67. Mock MB, Ringqvist I, Fisher LD, Davis KB, Chaitman BR, Kouchoukos NT, Kaiser GC, Alderman E, Ryan TJ, Russell RO, Jr., Mullin S, Fray D, Killip T, 3rd. Survival of medically treated patients in the coronary artery surgery study (CASS) registry. Circulation 1982;66(3):562–8.

68. Harris PJ, Harrell FE, Jr., Lee KL, Behar VS, Rosati RA. Survival in medically treated coronary artery disease. Circulation 1979;60(6):1259–69.

69. Hammermeister KE, DeRouen TA, Dodge HT. Evidence from a nonrandomized study that coronary surgery prolongs survival in patients with two-vessel coronary disease. Circulation 1979;59(3):430–5.

70. Elefteriades JA, Tolis G, Jr., Levi E, Mills LK, Zaret BL. Coronary artery bypass grafting in severe left ventricular dysfunction: excellent survival with improved ejection fraction and functional state. J Am Coll Cardiol 1993;22(5):1411–7.

71. Braunwald E, Rutherford JD. Reversible ischemic left ventricular dysfunction: evidence for the "hibernating myocardium". J Am Coll Cardiol 1986;8(6):1467–70.

72. Ragosta M, Beller GA, Watson DD, Kaul S, Gimple LW. Quantitative planar rest-redistribution 201Tl imaging in detection of myocardial viability and prediction of improvement in left ventricular function after coronary bypass surgery in patients with severely depressed left ventricular function. Circulation 1993;87(5):1630–41.

73. Mahrholdt H, Wagner A, Holly TA, Elliott MD, Bonow RO, Kim RJ, Judd RM. Reproducibility of chronic infarct size measurement by contrast-enhanced magnetic resonance imaging. Circulation 2002;106(18):2322–7.

74. Klein C, Nekolla SG, Bengel FM, Momose M, Sammer A, Haas F, Schnackenburg B, Delius W, Mudra H, Wolfram D, Schwaiger M. Assessment of myocardial viability with contrast-enhanced magnetic resonance imaging: comparison with positron emission tomography. Circulation 2002;105(2):162–7.

75. Fieno DS, Kim RJ, Chen EL, Lomasney JW, Klocke FJ, Judd RM. Contrast-enhanced magnetic resonance imaging of myocardium at risk: distinction between reversible and irreversible injury throughout infarct healing. J Am Coll Cardiol 2000;36(6):1985–91.

76. Kim RJ, Wu E, Rafael A, Chen EL, Parker MA, Simonetti O, Klocke FJ, Bonow RO, Judd RM. The use of contrast-enhanced magnetic resonance imaging to identify reversible myocardial dysfunction. N Engl J Med 2000;343(20):1445–53.

77. Gerber BL, Garot J, Bluemke DA, Wu KC, Lima JA. Accuracy of contrast-enhanced magnetic resonance imaging in predicting improvement of regional myocardial function in patients after acute myocardial infarction. Circulation 2002;106(9):1083–9.

78. Wellnhofer E, Olariu A, Klein C, Grafe M, Wahl A, Fleck E, Nagel E. Magnetic resonance low-dose dobutamine test is superior to scar quantification for the prediction of functional recovery. Circulation 2004;109(18):2172–4.

79. Kim RJ, Manning WJ. Viability assessment by delayed enhancement cardiovascular magnetic resonance: will low-dose dobutamine dull the shine? Circulation 2004;109(21):2476–9.

80. Amado LC, Kraitchman DL, Gerber BL, Castillo E, Boston RC, Grayzel J, Lima JA. Reduction of "no-reflow" phenomenon by intra-aortic balloon counterpulsation in a randomized magnetic resonance imaging experimental study. J Am Coll Cardiol 2004;43(7):1291–8.

81. Shan K, Constantine G, Sivananthan M, Flamm SD. Role of cardiac magnetic resonance imaging in the assessment of myocardial viability. Circulation 2004;109(11):1328–34.

82. Pennell DJ, Keegan J, Firmin DN, Gatehouse PD, Underwood SR, Longmore DB. Magnetic resonance imaging of coronary arteries: technique and preliminary results. Br Heart J 1993;70(4):315–26.

83. Manning WJ, Li W, Edelman RR. A preliminary report comparing magnetic resonance coronary angiography with conventional angiography. N Engl J Med 1993;328(12):828–32.

84. Pons Llado G. [Current state of non-invasive methods in the study of coronary arteries and surgical bypass grafts]. Rev Esp Cardiol 1998;51(7):510–20.

85. Weber OM, Martin AJ, Higgins CB. Whole-heart steady-state free precession coronary artery magnetic resonance angiography. Magn Reson Med 2003;50(6):1223–8.

86. Hofman MB, Wickline SA, Lorenz CH. Quantification of in-plane motion of the coronary arteries during the cardiac cycle: implications for acquisition window duration for MR flow quantification. J Magn Reson Imaging 1998;8(3):568–76.

87. Wang Y, Vidan E, Bergman GW. Cardiac motion of coronary arteries: variability in the rest period and implications for coronary MR angiography. Radiology 1999;213(3):751–8.

88. Bornert P, Stuber M, Botnar RM, Kissinger KV, Koken P, Spuentrup E, Manning WJ. Direct comparison of 3D spiral vs. Cartesian gradient-echo coronary magnetic resonance angiography. Magn Reson Med 2001;46(4):789–94.

89. Yang PC, Meyer CH, Terashima M, Kaji S, McConnell MV, Macovski A, Pauly JM, Nishimura DG, Hu BS. Spiral magnetic resonance coronary angiography with rapid real-time localization. J Am Coll Cardiol 2003;41(7):1134–41.

90. Deshpande VS, Shea SM, Laub G, Simonetti OP, Finn JP, Li D. 3D magnetization-prepared true-FISP: a new technique for imaging coronary arteries. Magn Reson Med 2001;46(3):494–502.

91. Huber ME, Paetsch I, Schnackenburg B, Bornstedt A, Nagel E, Fleck E, Boesiger P, Maggioni F, Cavagna FM, Stuber M. Performance of a new gadolinium-based intravascular contrast agent in free-breathing inversion-recovery 3D coronary MRA. Magn Reson Med 2003;49(1):115–21.

92. Kim WY, Danias PG, Stuber M, Flamm SD, Plein S, Nagel E, Langerak SE, Weber OM, Pedersen EM, Schmidt M, Botnar RM, Manning WJ. Coronary magnetic resonance angiography for the detection of coronary stenoses. N Engl J Med 2001;345(26):1863–9.

93. Ropers D, Baum U, Pohle K, Anders K, Ulzheimer S, Ohnesorge B, Schlundt C, Bautz W, Daniel WG, Achenbach S. Detection of coronary artery stenoses with thin-slice multidetector row spiral computed tomography and multiplanar reconstruction. Circulation 2003;107(5):664–6.

94. Leta R, Carreras F, Alomar X, Monell J, Garcia-Picart J, Auge JM, Salvador A, Pons-Llado G. Non-invasive coronary angiography with 16 multidetector-row spiral computed tomography: a comparative study with invasive coronary angiography. Rev Esp Cardiol 2004;57(3):217–24.

95. Hundley WG, Clarke GD, Landau C, Lange RA, Willard JE, Hillis LD, Peshock RM. Noninvasive determination of infarct artery patency by cine magnetic resonance angiography. Circulation 1995;91(5):1347–53.

96. Langerak SE, Kunz P, de Roos A, Vliegen HW, van Der Wall EE. Evaluation of coronary artery bypass grafts by magnetic resonance imaging. J Magn Reson Imaging 1999;10(3):434–41.

97. Langerak SE, Vliegen HW, de Roos A, Zwinderman AH, Jukema JW, Kunz P, Lamb HJ, van Der Wall EE. Detection of vein graft disease using high-resolution magnetic resonance angiography. Circulation 2002;105(3):328–33.

98. Constantine G, Shan K, Flamm SD, Sivananthan MU. Role of MRI in clinical cardiology. Lancet 2004;363(9427):2162–71.

99. Blackwell GG, Pohost GM. The evolving role of MRI in the assessment of coronary artery disease. Am J Cardiol 1995;75(11):74D-8D.

100. Kramer CM. Integrated approach to ischemic heart disease. The one-stop shop. Cardiol Clin 1998;16(2):267–76.

101. Botnar RM, Perez AS, Witte S, Wiethoff AJ, Laredo J, Hamilton J, Quist W, Parsons EC, Jr., Vaidya A, Kolodziej A, Barrett JA, Graham PB, Weisskoff RM, Manning WJ, Johnstone MT. In vivo molecular imaging of acute and subacute thrombosis using a fibrin-binding magnetic resonance imaging contrast agent. Circulation 2004;109(16):2023–9.

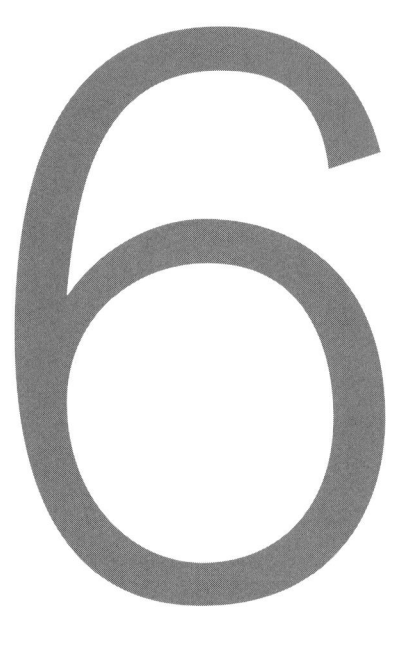

Cardiac and Paracardiac Masses

FRANCESC CARRERAS

6.1 Introduction

Primary cardiac tumors are a rare cause of heart disease, being found in autopsic series with a mean frequency of 0.02%, corresponding to 200 tumors in 1 million autopsies[1]. Three quarters of primary cardiac tumors are benign and the rest are malignant. Atrial myxoma, a benign neoplasm, is by far the most common primary cardiac tumor, while the majority of primary cardiac malignancies are angiosarcomas or rhabdomyosarcomas (Table 6.1). Cardiac metastases are 10 to 40 times more frequent than primary cardiac tumors, melanoma being the most common, although clinically undetected in a large percentage of cases. The diagnosis of a tumor involving the cardiovascular system in alive patients was difficult in the past due to the elusive character of clinical signs and symptoms, their recognition being usually made at post-mortem examinations.

Cardiac tumors or masses are frequently an unsuspected finding in asymptomatic patients. Their clinical manifestations, when present, are related to their localization, size or behavior, causing pericardial effusion (metastases, mesotheliomas), compression of the cavities (cysts, thymomas, lymphomas), myocardial restriction (fibromas, hemangiomas, sarcomas), paroxistic pulmonary or central venous congestion (myxomas), or peripheral embolism (thrombi, papillary fibroelastoma).

Although a first line diagnostic tool, echocardiography does have limitations: poor image quality in those cases with a difficult acoustic window, and limited field of view, especially in paracardiac masses. In the latter, the differential diagnosis is frequently challenging as extrinsic cardiac compression may be due to many different causes[2, 3], such as pleural efussion, hiatal hernia, or, simply, a chest wall malformation as in pectus excavatum. In all these situations, CMR is an excellent alternative imaging method (Figure 6.1). But also in the study of intracardiac masses CMR has become the preferred technique, due to its excellent image resolution and the possibility of obtaining angulated image planes, although in some aspects, as in the detection of calcifications, computed tomography is ahead[4]. Provided the variety of techniques available, a knowledge of their relative merits in the diagnosis of cardiac masses is important[5] (Table 6.2).

6.2 Technical Aspects in the Evaluation of Masses with CMR

The excellent soft tissue definition that CMR provides allows the clear delineation of the myocardium, pericardium, paracardiac fat, vascular structures, and the lungs, and thus facilitates the identification and study of abnormal masses. The wide field of view permits unlimited observation of the extension and the anatomical relationships of cardiac and paracardiac masses with the great vessels and the bronchial tree, information that is espe-

cially useful to guide surgeons in the design of an appropriate therapeutical strategy[6,7].

To some extent, CMR allows some degree of tumor tissue characterization[8] by a comparative analysis of signal intensity characteristics on the images from the different sequences available (Table 6.3). Easy to characterize are those tumors with a high fat content, such as lipomas[9], which stand out for their bright signal intensity in T1w spin-echo (SE) sequences (Figure 6.2). Comparing the characteristics of the same image in T1w and T2w SE sequences, the composition of an

Table 6.1 Classification of the most frequent masses and cardiac tumors

Primary		Secondary		
Benign	Malignant	Direct extension	Venous extension	Metastatic extension
Myxoma	Sarcoma	Lung carcinoma	Renal cell carcinoma	Melanoma
Pericardial cyst	Mesothelioma	Breast carcinoma	Adrenal carcinoma	Leukemia
Lipoma	Lymphoma	Esophageal carcinoma	Hepatocellular carcinoma	Lymphoma
Fibroelastoma		Mediastinal tumors	Thyroid carcinoma	Genitourinary tract
Rhabdomyoma			Carcinoma of the lung	Gastrointestinal tract
Fibroma			Sarcoma of the uterus	
Hemangioma				

FIGURE 6.1

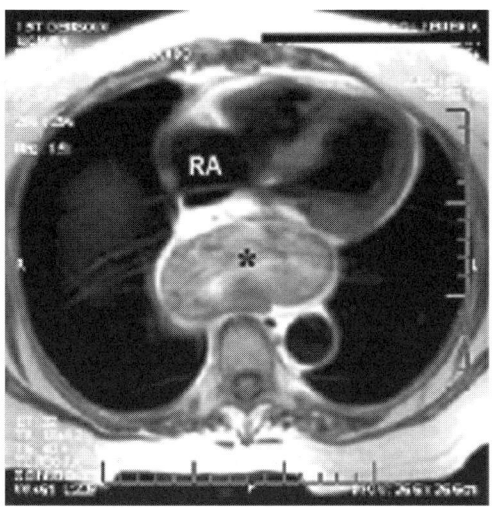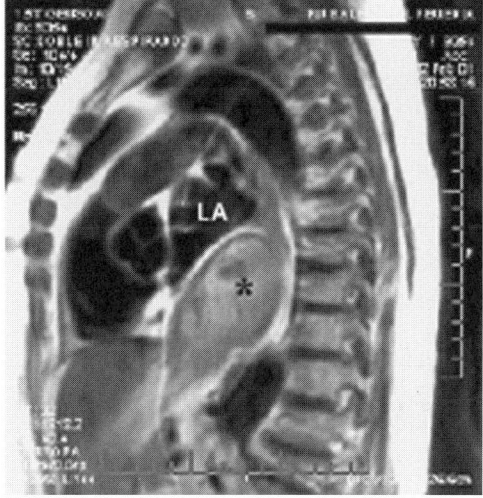

F. 6.1. Axial (left) and sagittal (right) images showing a large hiatal hernia (asterisks) compressing the posterior aspect of the heart. LA: left atrium; RA: right atrium.

Table 6.2 Usefulness of different diagnostic techniques for the study of cardiac tumors*

	x-ray	CT scan	Angiography	Echocardiography	CMR
Primary benign					
Myxoma	+	+++	++	++++	+++
Pericardial cyst	++	+++	0	+	++++
Lipoma	0	++	0	+++	++++
Fibroelastoma	0	++	0	++++	++
Rhabdomyoma	0	++	+	+++	++++
Fibroma	0	+++	+	+++	++++
Primary malignant					
Sarcoma	+	+++	+	+++	++++
Mesothelioma	+	+++	+	++	++++
Lymphoma	++	+++	+	++	++++
Secondary tumors					
Direct proliferation	+	+++	++	+++	++++
Vein proliferation	0	+++	+++	+++	++++
Metastases	+	+++	+	++	++++

0: not useful; +: occasionally useful; ++: usually provides some information; +++ always useful; ++++: prefered diagnostic test.* Modified from Salcedo et al[5].

Table 6.3 Basical differential diagnosis of a cardiac mass according to signal intensity characteristics

- *High on T1w SE*: fat, effect of paramagnetic contrast, recent subacute hemorrhage (1 to 3 days)
- *Intermediate on T1w and high on T2w SE*: tumor, thrombus, cyst with elevated protein content
- *Low in T1w and very high on T2w SE*: serous cyst
- *Intermediate on GRE*: tumor
- *Low on GRE*: Thrombus or a mass with a high iron content

effusion or cyst can be assessed (Figure 6.3), although it should be noted that the signal of the hematic collections varies according to the degree of hemoglobin decomposition related to time (Table 6.4). This information is useful for the approximate dating of the evolution time of an hematoma[10] (Figure 6.4). Masses and tumors with a high iron content presents with an intermediate signal intensity on T1w SE and low signal intensity on gradient-echo (GRE) imaging. This characteristic is useful to diferentiate a thrombus (Figure 6.5) from a mass of another origin. The presence of hemorrhage or necrosis within the tumor can characteristically alter its appearance (Figure 6.6). On the other hand, intravenous administration of paramagnetic contrast agents permits to estimate the degree of vascularization of the mass (Figures 6.6 and 6.7), this helping in the identification of intramyocardial masses[11].

A complete scanning protocol of cardiac and paracardiac masses should include axial, coronal and sagittal multislice T1w and T2w SE or turbo SE images, a multislice axial T1w SE acquisition after administration of gadolinium-DTPA, and finally a cine GRE sequence in the plane of the cardiac mass, which is very useful in assessing tumor motion.

In practice, the decision to use CMR for the evaluation of a cardiac or paracardiac mass is almost always based on a previous echocardiogram in which the presence of an abnormal mass was suspected. Although CMR will always be helpful in assessing the location, anatomical relations and characterization of the lesion, in our experience, differentiation between benign and malignant cardiac tumors by their signal characteristics is usually disappointing, as some studies have confirmed[12].

6.3 Malignant Primary Cardiac Tumors

Malignant neoplasms are classified by tissue type as mesenchimal (sarcoma), lymphoid (lymphoma), and mesothelial (mesothe-

Table 6.4 Signal intensity (SI) of an hemorrhage related to time and to type of hemoglobin

Condition	Hemoglobin	T1w SE SI	T2w SE SI
Acute (<24 hours)	Oxyhemoglobin	Intermediate	Intermediate
Recent subacute (1–3 days)	Deoxyhemoglobin	High*	Intermediate
Late subacute (3–14 days)	Metahemoglobin	Intermediate**	High
Chronic subacute (>14 days)	Hemosiderin***	Low	Low

*Homogeneous signal

**Heterogeneous signal (intermediate/high)

***The accumulation of hemosiderin produces a very low or even absent SI.

FIGURE 6.2

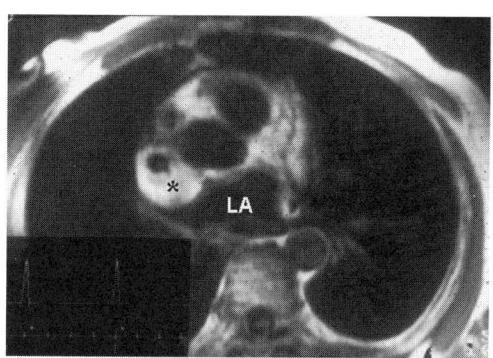

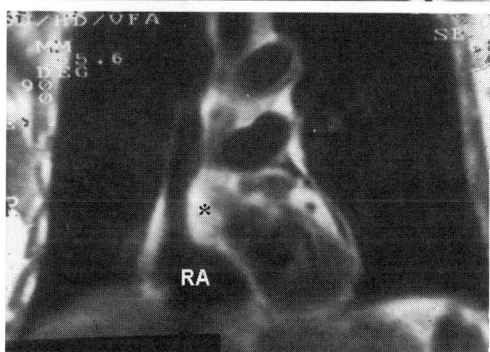

FIGURE 6.3

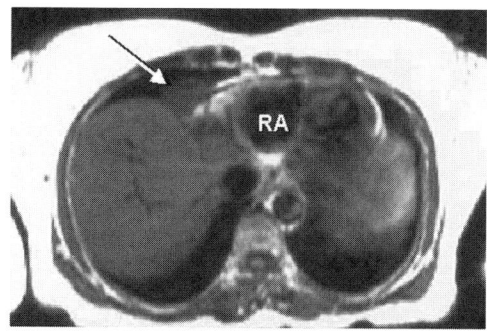

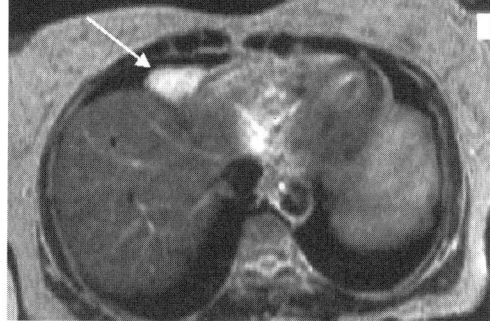

FIGURE 6.4

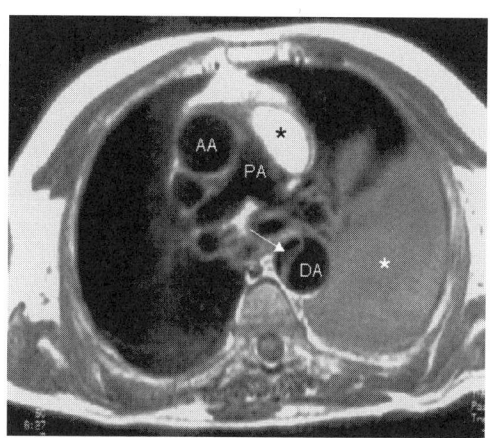

F. 6.2. T1w SE axial (top) and coronal (bottom) images depicting a lipoma (asterisk) involving the superior segment of the interatrial septum and the superior vena cava. LA: left atrium; RA: right atrium.

F. 6.3. Axial T1w SE (top) and T2w SE (bottom) images from a pericardial cyst adjacent to the right atrium (RA): observe the low signal intensity on T1w SE, that increases substantially on T2w SE, indicating fluid contents of the mass.

F. 6.4. Axial T1w SE sequence in a case of acute dissection of the aorta (arrow) showing mediastinal hematoma (black asterisk) and left hemothorax (white asterisk); the high intensity of the hematoma suggests a recent subacute event, while the intermeditate signal of the hemothorax indicates, in turn, late subacute effusion (see Table 6.4). AA: ascending aorta; DA: descending aorta; PA: pulmonary artery.

FIGURE 6.5

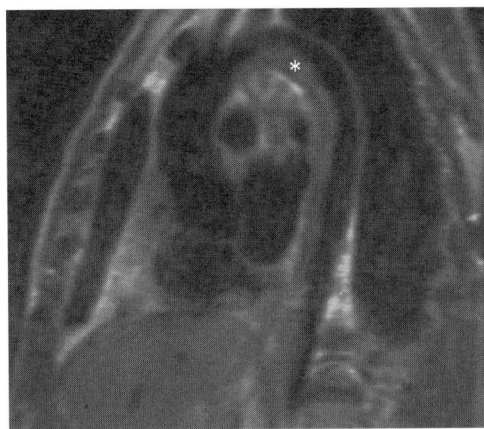
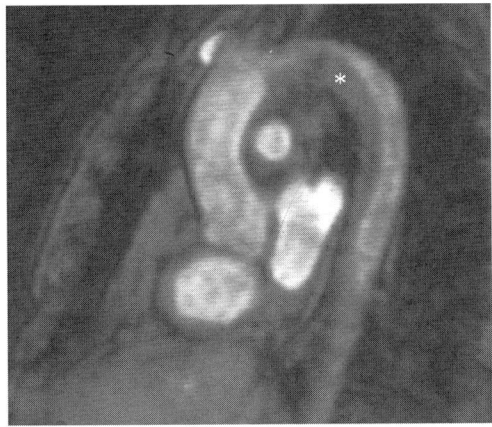

FIGURE 6.6

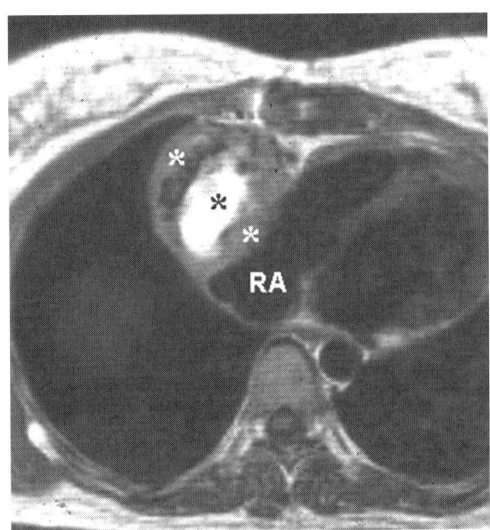
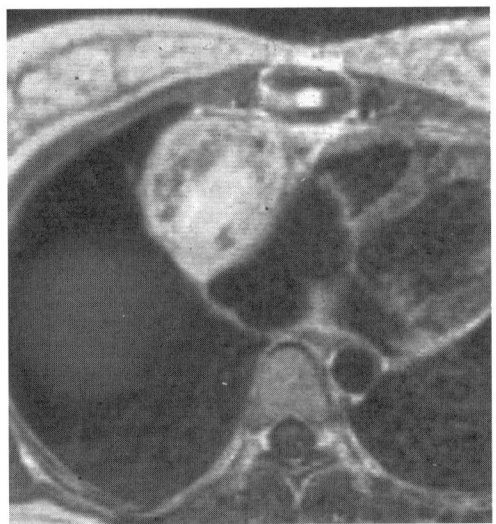

FIGURE 6.7

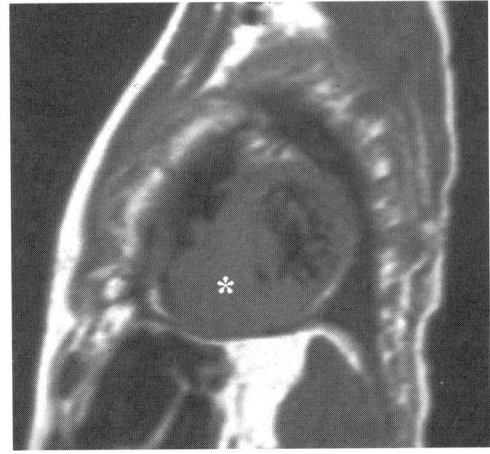
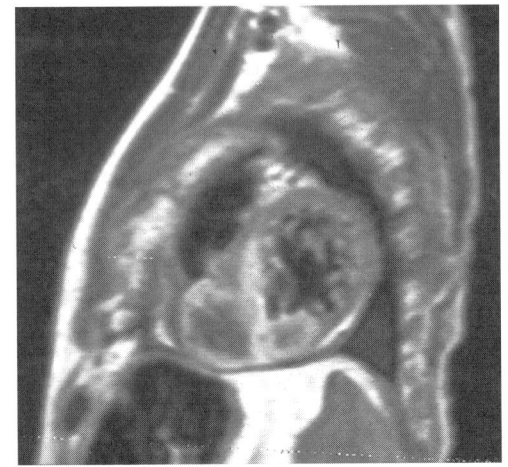

lioma)[13]. Sarcomas are the most frequent malignancies of this group.

a. Angiosarcoma

Angiosarcomas are one of the most common mesenchimal tumors in surgical studies and occur slightly more often in middle-aged males. Because they tend to locate at the right atrium[14], occlusion of the inflow from the caval veins, or obstruction of the right ventricular outflow tract may occur. Also, as the pericardium is frequently involved, patients usually present with pericarditis, right-sided heart failure or tamponade[15].

Figure 6.6 corresponds to a patient that presented with symptoms of acute pericarditis, affected by an angiosarcoma that appeared as an intramural mass of the right atrial wall with pericardial infiltration. The patient underwent surgery, the tumor was resected and the right atrial wall was reconstructed using a pericardium patch (Figure 6.8). The clinical follow-up was in accordance with other cases described in the literature[16] as the patient died a few months following surgery due to disseminate metastases.

b. Myxosarcoma

The diagnosis of atrial myxosarcoma is difficult for the pathologist and sometimes can be erroneously diagnosed as a myxoma[17]. The case in Figure 6.9 happened to a young patient in whom an intraventricular mass had been diagnosed by echocardiography, without evidence of metases on the systemic exam. An intraoperative direct biopsy of the tumor was not conclusive for malignancy, suggesting a diagnosis of myxoma, and the mass was surgically removed. Because of the involvement of mitral valve apparatus, the mitral valve was also resected and a metallic prosthesis implanted. However, a detailed pathologic exam of the whole excised mass demonstrated the presence of myxosarcoma. The image presented in Figure 6.9 corresponds to a relapse of the tumor a few months later.

6.4 Benign Primary Cardiac Tumors

Benign neoplasms are usually classified pathologically according to histologic features and cellular differentiation. The differential diagnosis of malignant from benign tumors with imaging techniques is usually difficult, since there are no specific differential characteristics. Nevertheless, it has been mentioned that a benign lesion tipically presents with an homogenous signal intensity at CMR, is located at the left heart and is not associated with pleural or pericardial effusion[12] (Figure 6.10). The homogenous character of benign lesions is due to the fact that they grow slowly, while malignant tumors, which grow rapidly, normally contain foci of hemorrhage or necrosis giving an heterogeneous signal intensity. However, this is not always the rule, as in the case of hemangiomas, benign tumors with an important vascular component (Figure 6.11).

a. Myxoma

Myxomas are the most frequent primary cardiac neoplasms, endocardial-based masses not infiltrating the underlying tissues.

F. 6.5. Oblique sagittal views oriented on the plane of the thoracic aorta. An extense mural thrombus of the aorta is seen (asterisk) with an intermediate signal intensity on the T1w SE sequence (left) and rather low signal intensity on GRE (right).

F. 6.6. At left: T1w SE image of an intramural tumor involving the wall of the right atrium (RA). Two components are distinguished in the tumor mass: one with a non-homogeneous low to intermediate signal intensity (white asterisks), and a nuclear zone exhibiting very high signal intensity (black asterisk), suggestive of recent hemorrhage. At right: Substantial increase in signal intensity of the peripheral component is seen after gadolinium administration proving its densely vascularized character. The tumor proved to be an hemangiosarcoma at surgery.

F. 6.7. Left: T1w SE sagittal view oriented on the short-axis of the ventricles: there is a large increase in thickness of the posterior interventricular septum (asterisk), which bulges into the right ventricular cavity, the intensity signal at this level being apparently uniform. Right: the same sequence is shown after the administration of gadolinium: the increase in signal intensity is highly heterogenous, proving that there are areas with different degrees of vascularization within the mass. The case corresponded to a myocardial metastatic tumor.

FIGURE 6.8

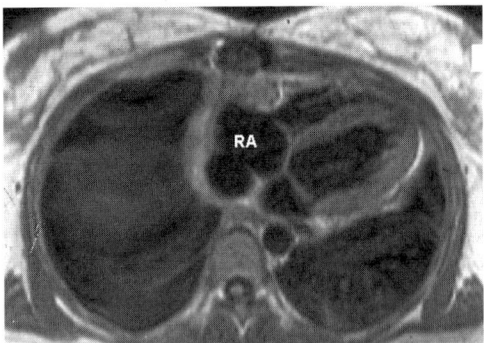

FIGURE 6.9

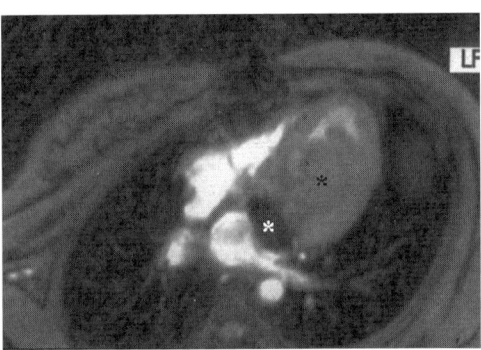

FIGURE 6.10

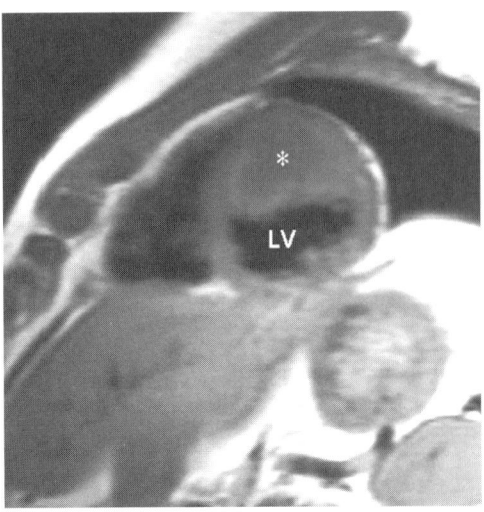

FIGURE 6.11

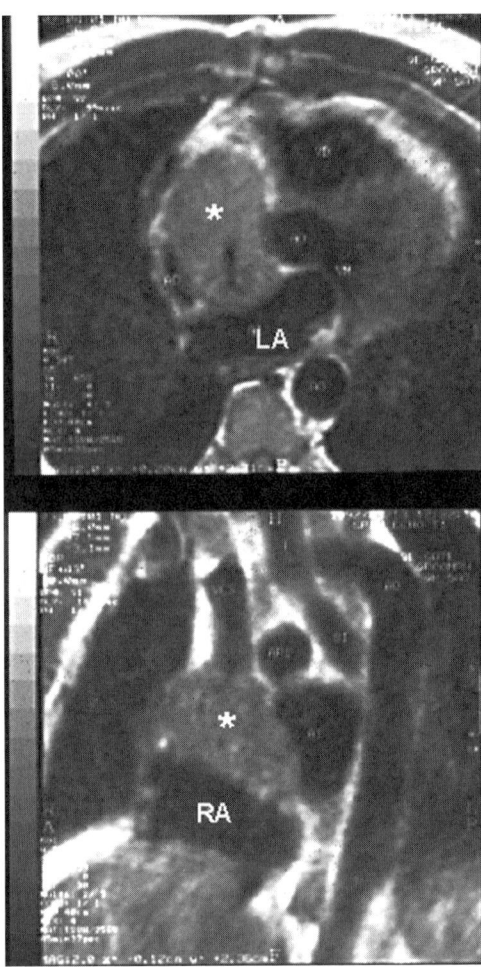

F. 6.8. Axial T1w SE plane obtained from the same patient presented in Figure 6.6 after a tumor resection and reconstruction of the wall of the right atrium (RA) were performed.

F. 6.9. Axial GRE showing a large sesile intraventricular uniform mass (black asterisk) corresponding to a recurrence of a previously excised myxosarcoma. Note the artifact induced by a mechanical mitral valve prosthesis (white asterisk).

F. 6.10. Fast SE sequence on a short-axis plane of the left ventricle (LV) showing an homogeneous intramural mass (asterisk) protruding into the ventricular chamber. The case corresponds to a young, asymptomatic patient that refused further investigations. Although the etiology of the process remains uncertain, most CMR features do certainly correspond to a bening tumor: uniform signal of the mass, location at the left heart, and absence of pericardial or pleural effusion.

F. 6.11. T1w SE images in axial (top) and sagittal (bottom) planes of a benign hemangioma (asterisk) occupying a large part of the right atrium (RA) and displaying a slightly heterogeneous intensity signal due to its vascular structure. LA: left atrium.

Although the majority of myxomas are attached to the endocardium by a broad-based or pedunculated stalk, approximately one-fourth are sessile[18]. Although the vast majority attach at the fosa ovalis of the interatrial septum (Figure 6.12), they can arise anywhere from the endocardial surface[19] (Figure 6.13). Cine gradient-echo images may display their point of attachment and their swinging motion if they are pedunculated. Their signal intensity may be heterogeneous due to their myxomatous components and calcifications that appear low on T1w and high on T2w images[20]. Subacute hemorrage areas display a high signal intensity in both T1w and T2w images, while fresh hemorrages have intermediate to low signal intensity on T1w and low signal intensity on T2w images[21]. Their signal intensity enhances after gadolinium administration, usually with an heterogeneous pattern[22].

b. Fibroma

Cardiac fibroma is a congenital neoplasm that typically affects children, and is the pediatric cardiac tumor most commonly resected. However, 15% of cardiac fibromas occur in adolescents and adults[23]. They are well-circumscribed tumors located within the ventricular myocardium (Figure 6.14). At CMR imaging fibromas usually appear as a discrete mural mass, with slightly low signal intensity on T1w SE and well defined edges, which is useful to distinguish fibromas from hypertrophic cardiomyopathy (Figure 6.15). When the mass is usually isointense relative to the myocardium on T1w images, T2w SE sequence can be helpful for its detection, as it appears hypointense because of the fibrous tissue. The involved myocardium shows reduced contractility on cine GRE sequences. Contrast-enhanced imaging may help to delineate the boundaries of the tumor, although the signal is heterogeneous and not very intense due to its poor vascularization[24].

c. Lipoma

Lipomas are the most frequently diagnosed benign tumors[25]. They are generally found in the interatrial septal wall (Figure 6.16), and their diagnosis is usually suspected based on a previous echocardiographic study. Although multislice CT scanning has demonstrated to be a useful technique for the recognition of the lipomatous hypertrophy of the interatrial septum[9], including its characterization as fatty according to its signal intensity (-150 to -50 Hounsfield units), CMR is the prefered diagnostic technique due to its capability to clearly detect the fatty composition of the tumor, as fat is characteristically depicted as a bright intense signal.

d. Pericardial masses and tumors

The most frequent benign disorders are pericardial cysts[26] (see chapter 7), which, depending on their location, can cause hemodynamic compromise (Figure 6.17). Cysts show a low intensity signal on T1w SE and high signal intensity on T2w, although if they contain a high amount of fibrin or blood, the T1w signal can be of an intermediate or high signal intensity.

An exceptional case in our series is that of a patient who presented with an intrapericardial mass of relatively homogeneous characteristics, with intermediate signal intensity on T1w, increasing heterogeneously on T2w (Figure 6.18), and compressing the right ventricle. The mass was surgically removed and turned out to be a large fibrin aggregate in the pericardial cavity.

6.5 Secondary Cardiac Tumors

Secondary cardiac tumors have an incidence of up to 1% at necropsy, 20 times more common than are primary tumors[27]. Metastatic disease may result from contiguous extension, lymphangitic spread, or hematogenous spread[28]. Although clinically silent in the majority of cases, cardiac metastases usually present in the form of a large pericardial effusion or cardiac tamponade[29].

a. Mediastinal lymphomas

Malignant hematological processes involving the mediastinum are the most frequent cases of this group, lymphomas in particular[30], which give rise to a mass of homogeneous characteristics of intermediate density that increase with the administration of gadolinium. Mediastinal infiltration is usually extensive, frequently involving the vascular structures, either by

FIGURE 6.12

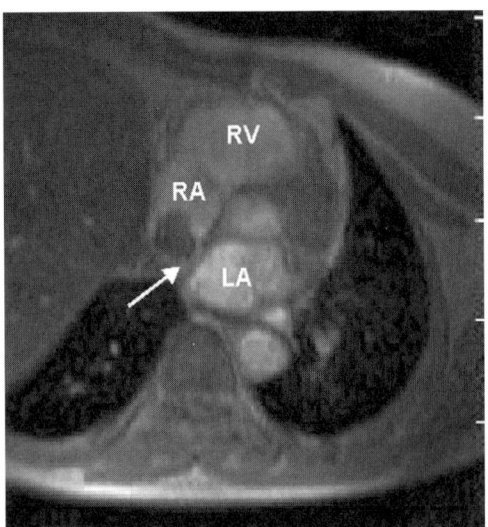

FIGURE 6.13

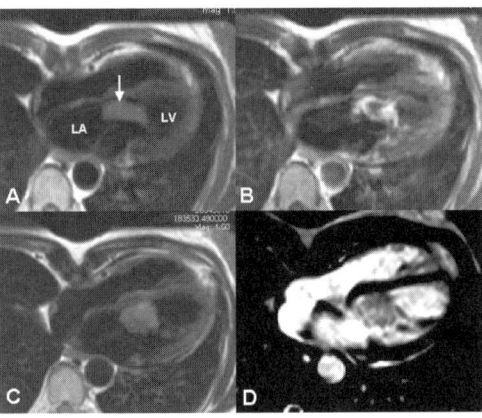

FIGURE 6.14

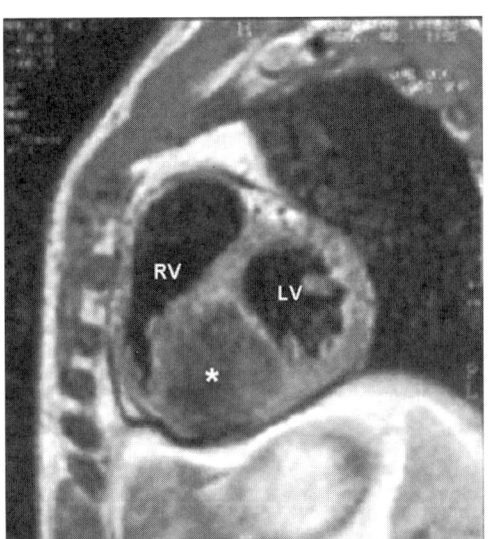

FIGURE 6.15

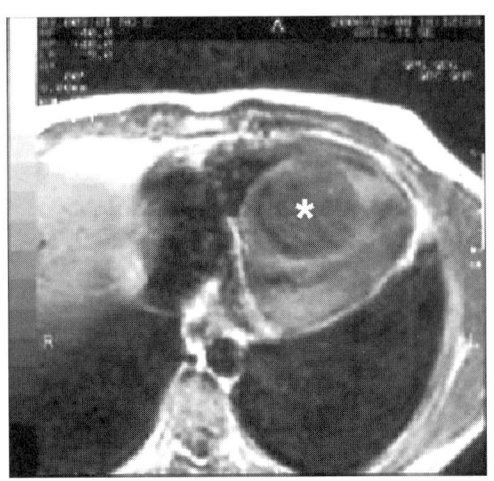

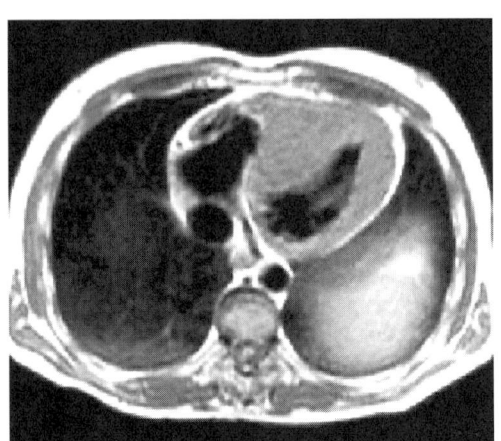

FIGURE 6.16

FIGURE 6.17

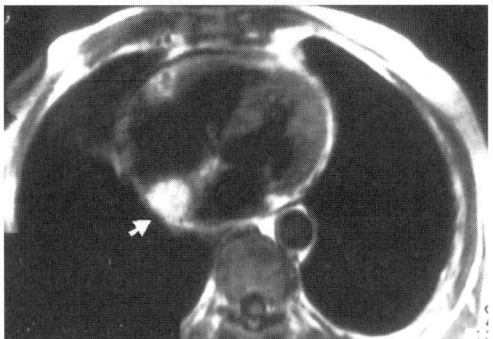

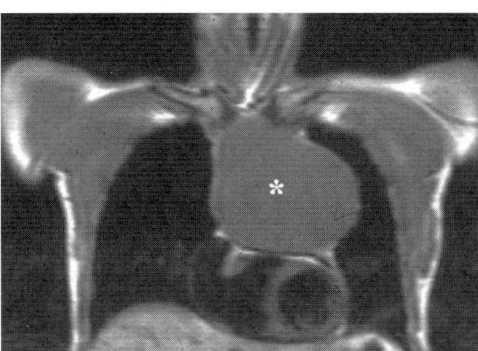

FIGURE 6.18

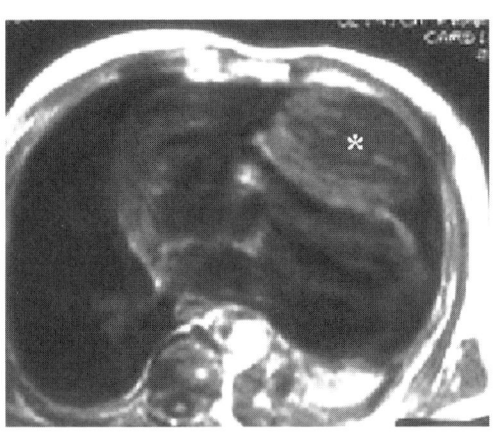

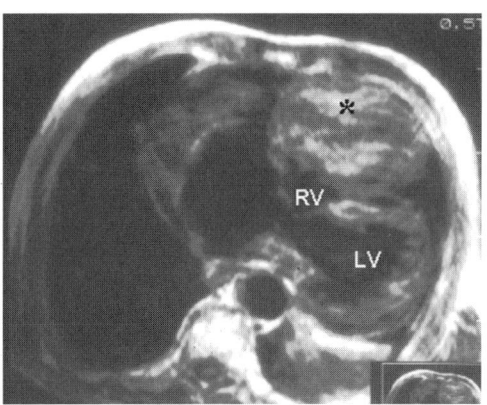

F. 6.12. Axial GRE image showing a myxoma attached by a pediculum (arrow) to the right aspect of the interatrial septum. LA: left atrium; RA: righ atrium; RV: right ventricle.

F. 6.13. Myxoma attached to the mitral annulus, at the base of the anterior leaflet shown on T1w SE (A), T1w SE with gadolinium (B), T2w SE (C) and GRE (D).

F. 6.14. T1w SE oblique sagittal view showing an intramural mass (asterisk) with low signal intensity that involves the interventricular septum, its borders being well defined, without infiltrating the myocardium. This process was found in an asymptomatic young patient who has refused further investigations for years, the mass having the characteristical features of a benign myocardial fibroma.

F. 6.15. Axial T1w SE sequence (left) from the same patient that in Figure 6.16, showing slightly lower signal intensity than the surrounding myocardium and defined boundaries of the intramural mass at the septal level, which are useful signs to distinguish the process from a hypertrophic cardiomyopathy (right), sometimes exhibiting similar degrees of wall thickness although with uniform signal intensity within the myocardium.

F. 6.16. Axial T1w SE showing a lipoma located at the interatrial septum (arrow).

F. 6.17. Coronal T1w SE in a patient with a giant pericardial cyst (asterisk) located at the anterior superior mediastinum and compressing the cardiac chambers.

F. 6.18. Large intrapericardial mass with well-defined borders, presenting with low to intermediate signal intensity on T1w SE (white asterisk, at left), that increases heterogeneously on T2w SE (black asterisk, at right). Observe the compression of the right ventricle (RV) by the mass, which prompted its surgical removal, this proving the mass to be an organized fibrin aggregate. LV: left ventricle.

infiltration or by compression. Cardiovascular involvement can be manifested in different ways. When the superior mediastinum is predominantly involved, superior vena cava compression is frequent (Figure 6.19), leading to a characteristic collar-shaped edema of the superior half of the chest. If the process involves the posterior mediastinum, compression of the left atrium and the pulmonary veins is observed (Figure 6.20). A compression of the right atrium and an involvement of the pericardium can be seen when the lymphoma is located in the anterior mediastinum (Figure 6.21).

Retroperitoneal fibrosis with mediastinal involvement is a rare condition that must be distinguished from lymphomas. Figure 6.22 presents the case of a patient with this condition, which is less aggresive than lymphoma. The fibrotic mass surrounds the abdominal aorta and spreads to the mediastinum traversing the diaphragm. The progression of the mass surrounds intramediastinal large vessels and the heart, infiltrating the right atrial wall and the anterior pericardium.

b. Lung carcinoma

Lung carcinomas can cause compression or, more frequently, infiltration (Figure 6.23) of the cardiac structures by direct extension, and on occasions they may infiltrate the left atrium via the pulmonary veins (Figure 6.24).

c. Melanoma

Malignant melanoma has the highest rate of cardiac metastases, as cardiac involvement postmortem is found in approximately half of the cases of disseminated melanoma, affecting all the chambers of the heart. This finding is made with increasing frequency because of the improving survival of patients with melanoma[31]. Cardiac metastases can present as a lobulated mass filling the ventricular cavity, adherent to and infiltrating the myocardium. The anatomic site and the extent of tumor growth are important factors and magnetic resonance images of the mass are helpful in determining the surgical procedure[32].

d. Pericardial secondary tumors

Malignant tumors involving the pericardium most commonly represent direct extension of regional disease or metastasic spread from breast and lung carcinomas, melanomas, leukemia and lymphoma[26], and are much more frequent than primary tumors (mesothelioma). In cases of direct extension, a loss of the normal continuity of the pericardium, abnormal pericardial thickening or the presence of an effusion are observed using CMR (Figure 6.25). In hematogenous dissemination, focal involvement due to nodular lesions, enlargement or also effusion, nearly always hemorrhagic, are usually observed.

6.6 Benign Paracardiac Masses or Pseudotumors

Although the majority of these processes are first detected by echocardiography, frequently is not possible to establish a precise diagnosis and, thus, CMR is always indicated. These are some examples from our experience:

- Masses of a vascular origin, such as a pseudoaneurysm of the aortic root appeared after an episode of aortic prothetic endocarditis (Figure 6.26), which was diagnosed by transesophageal echocardiography but not appropriately delimited until a CMR exam was performed. This information was useful to the surgeon, who decided not to resect but to seal its connection with the aorta by means of a teflon patch.
- Enlargement of cardiac silhouette not due to a pericardial effusion but rather to large subepicardial lipoma (Figure 6.27). These disorders are usually detected with echocardiography and, according to the clinical situation of the patient, may be confused with an efussion or an infiltrating mass of the pericardium, such as a lymphoma.
- Deformation and/or compression of the cardiac structures due to a diaphragmatic hernia (Figure 6.1), a pectus excavatum or to the presence of abdominal structures in the chest (Figure 6.28).

6.7 Intracavitary Thrombi

The diagnosis of an intracavitary thrombus is usually suspected from echocardiographic find-

FIGURE 6.19

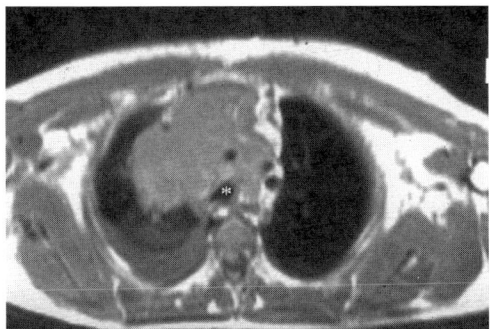

FIGURE 6.21

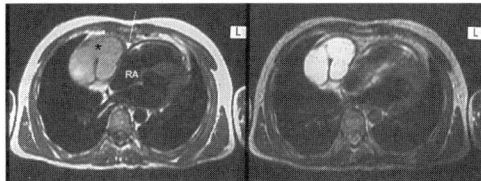

FIGURE 6.20

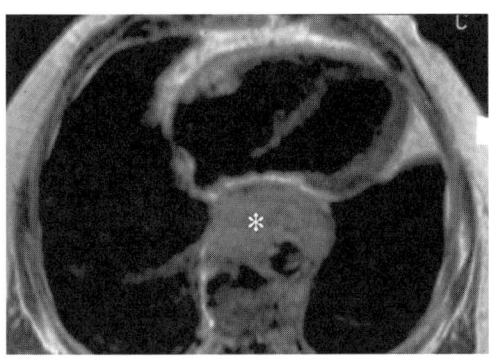 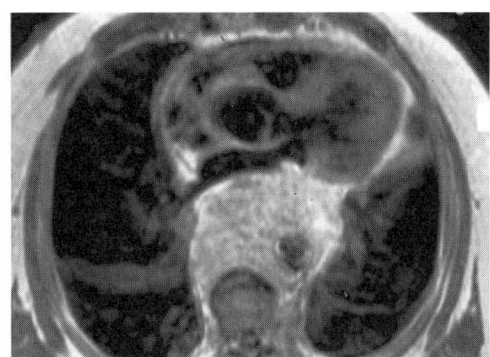

FIGURE 6.22

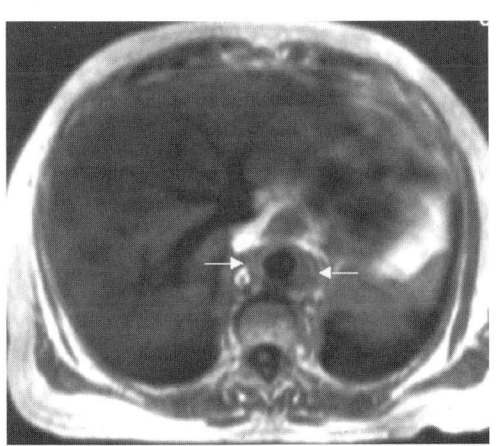 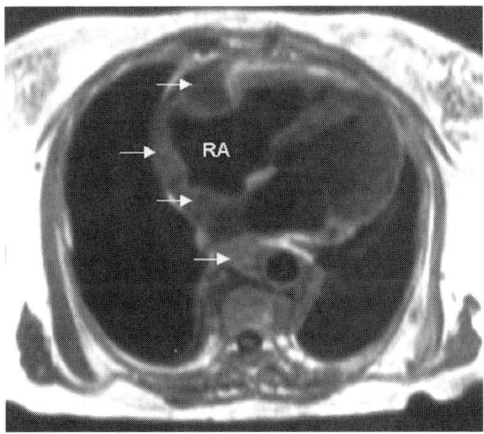

F. 6.19.   Axial T1w SE image from a patient with a mediastinal lymphoma compressing the trachea (asterisks) and the vessels of the superior mediastinum.

F. 6.20.   Axial T1w SE sequences before (left) and after (right) the administration of gadolinium: a large, well-defined, homogeneous, vascularized mass is seen on the posterior mediastinum compressing the structures of the heart. A transparietal biopsy gave the diagnosis of lymphoma.

F. 6.21.   Axial T1w (left) and T2w (right) SE images of a right paracardiac lymphoma that infiltrates the pericardium, with loss of continuity of the hypointense pericardial line (arrow). Note the increase in signal intensity in the T2w sequence. RA: right atrium.

F. 6.22.   Axial T1W SE images corresponding to a case of retroperitoneal fibrosis with medastinal involvement. Left panel: the fibrotic mass is observed surrounding the abdominal aorta (arrow). Right panel: the mediastinal involvement follows the course of the main vessels and infiltrates the wall of the right atrium (RA), the interatrial septum and the anterior pericardium (arrows).

FIGURE 6.23

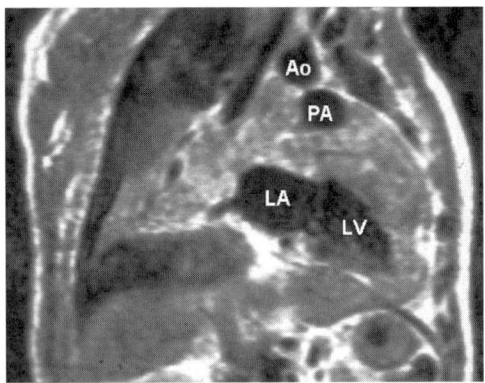

FIGURE 6.24

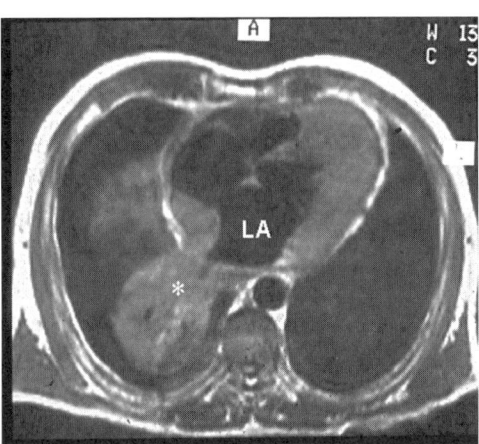

FIGURE 6.25

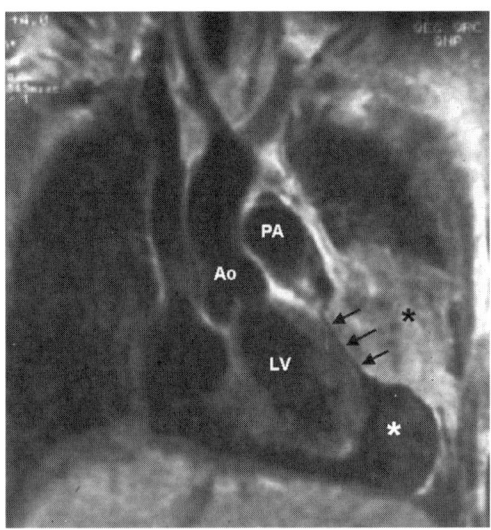

FIGURE 6.26

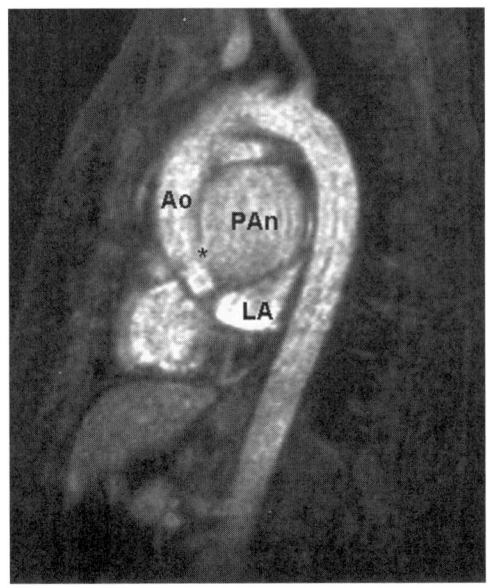

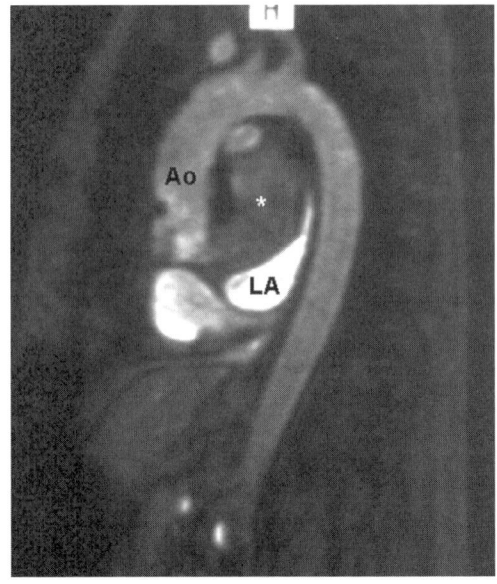

FIGURE 6.27

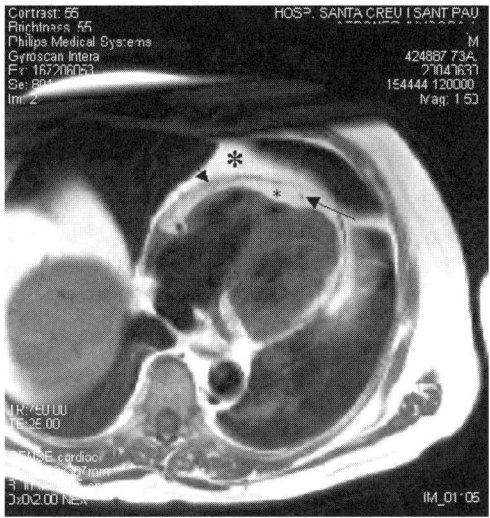 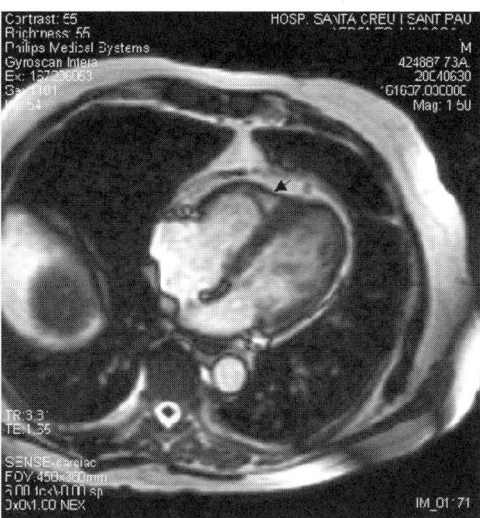

F. 6.23. Oblique sagittal T1w SE oriented on the vertical long axis of the left ventricle showing a huge increase in myocardial thickness due to infiltration from a lung carcinoma that makes heart chambers almost unrecognizable. Ao: aorta; LA: left atrium; LV: left ventricle; PA: pulmonary artery.

F. 6.24. Axial T1w SE in a case of lung carcinoma (asterisk) that infiltrates the heart through the right pulmonary veins and the left atrium (LA).

F. 6.25. Coronal T1w SE image from a patient with a left pulmonary lymphoma (black asterisk) involving the pericardium by continuity: there is a large pericardial effusion (white asterisk) and areas of pericardial infiltration by the tumor, where both the visceral an parietal layers are adhered (arrows). Ao: aorta; LV: left ventricle; PA: pulmonary artery.

F. 6.26. Oblique sagittal fast segmented GRE images showing, on the left panel, a large post-endocarditis aortic pseudoaneurysm (PAn) in communication (black asterisk) with the aorta (Ao), and compressing the left atrium (LA), the high signal intensity within the PAn indicating free flow within this cavity. On the right panel, after surgical exclusion, the PAn appears reduced in size and with a reduced intensity signal (white asterisk).

F. 6.27. Axial Fast SE (left) in a patient with profuse paracardiac adiposis; signals corresponding to the pericardium (short arrow) and the left anterior descending coronary artery (long arrow) help in the distinction between epicardial (small asterisk) and mediastinal (large asterisk) fat, which is characterized by a hyperintense signal. A Fast GRE sequence (right) shows also high intensity signal from fat, that contrasts sharply with that from the myocardium (arrow).

ings, in a patient with a predisposing clinical context. However, they can also be detected by CMR (see also chapter 5). Features of intracavitari thrombi may be very similar to those from a tumoral mass, at least on T1w SE images (Figure 6.29). On the other hand, the presence of blood flow artifacts can be confused with intracavitary masses, especially in those areas of slow blood flow or flow stasis[33]. The differential diagnosis is facilitated by observing whether or not the suspect image persists in different study image planes and by taking cine GRE sequences (Cine Loops 6.1 and 6.2 on CD; see also Cine Loop 5.12 on CD). Alternatively, MR tagging may help to distinguish between sluggish blood and throm-

bus[34]. Due to its high iron content, it is characteristic that the thrombus signal in the GRE images is of a very low intensity (dark) (Figure 6.30), standing out against the high intensity of the flow signal (bright), while the tumors usually present with an intermediate heterogeneous signal. It should be kept in mind, nevertheless, that myxomas also have a high iron content and, therefore, can have an appearance similar to the thrombi[35]. The cine sequence also allows to differentiate thrombus from flow artifacts if it is possible to identify the presence of defined mass edges. The use of a gadolinium-based paramagnetic contrasts also aids in the differential diagnosis between a tumor and a thrombus.

FIGURE 6.28

FIGURE 6.30

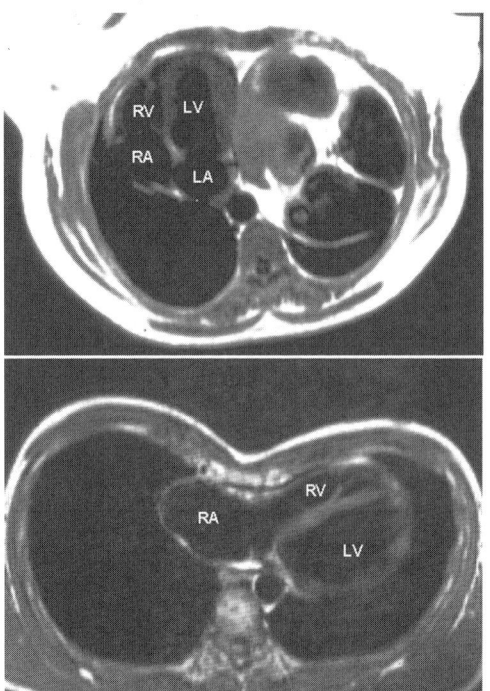

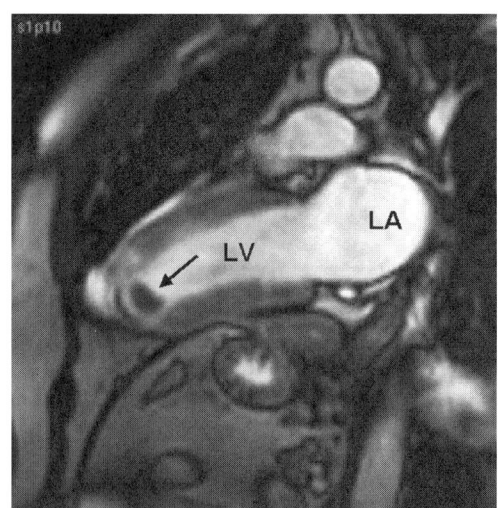

FIGURE 6.29

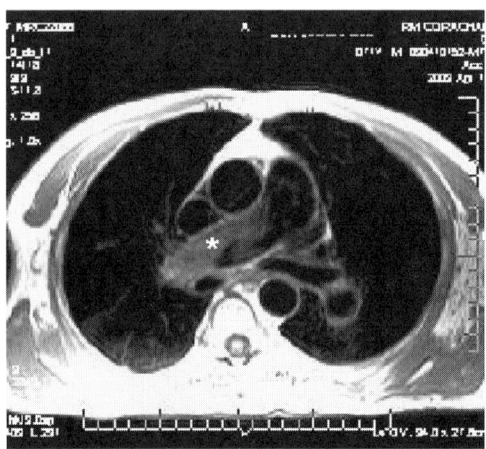

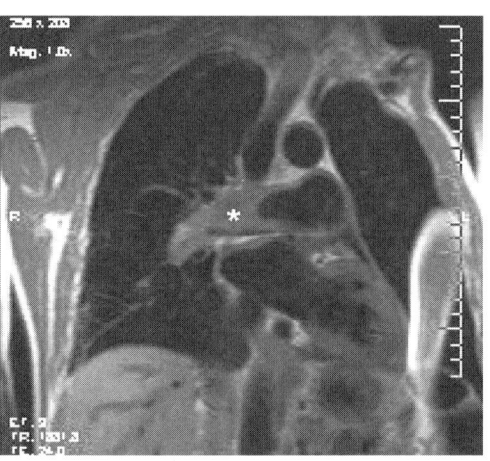

F. 6.28. Top: displacement of the heart to the right hemithorax due to a prominent left diaphragmatic paralysis with protrusion of the colon into the left hemithorax. Bottom: pectus excavatum with compression of the anterior aspect of the heart. LA: left atrium; LV: left ventricle; RA: right atrium; RV: right ventricle.

F. 6.29. Axial (left) and coronal (right) T1w SE sequences in a patient with an extensive thromboembolism (asterisk) of the right pulmonary artery.

F. 6.30. Frame from a cine sequence on a vertical long axis of the left ventricle (LV) in a patient with an antero-apical aneurysm and a mural thrombus (arrow); LA: left atrium.

References

1. Reynen K. Frequency of primary tumors of the heart. Am J Cardiol 1996;77:107

2. Brown JJ, Barakos JA, Higgins CB. Magnetic resonance imaging of cardiac and paracardiac masses. J Thorac Imag 1989; 4:58.

3. Menegus MA, Greenberg MA, Spindola-Franco H, Fayemi A. Magnetic resonance imaging of suspected atrial tumors. Am Heart J 1992; 123:1260–1268.

4. Grebenc ML, Rosado de Christenson M, Burke AP, Green CE, Galvin JR. Primary cardiac and pericardial neoplasms: radiologic-pathological correlation. Radiographics 2000; 1073–103.

5. Salcedo EE, Cohen GE, White RD, Davison MB. Cardiac tumors: diagnosis and management. Curr Probl Cardiol 1992; 17:73–137.

6. Murphy MC, Sweeney MS, Putnam JB Jr, Walker WE, Frazier OH, Ott DA, Cooley DA. Surgical treatment of cardiac tumors: a 25-year experience. Ann Thorac Surg 1990; 49:612–618.

7. Lundt JT, Ehman RL, Julsrud PR, et al. Cardiac masses: assessment by MR imaging. Am J Roentgenol 1989; 152:469–473.

8. Semelka RC, Shoenut JP, Wilson ME, Pellech AE, Patton JN. Cardiac masses: signal intensity features on SE, gradient-echo, gadolinium-enhanced SE, and turboFLASH images. J Magn Reson Imaging 1992; 2:415–420.

9. Heyer CM, Kagel T, Lemburg SP, Bauer TT, Nicolas V. Lipomatous hypertrophy of the interatrial septum. Chest 2003; 124:2068–73.

10. Seelos KC, Funari M, Chang JM, Higgins CB. Magnetic resonance imaging in acute and subacute mediastinal bleeding. Am Heart J 1992; 123:1269–1272.

11. Funari M, Fujita N, Peck WW, Higgins CB. Cardiac tumors: assessment with Gd-DTPA enhanced imaging. J Comput Assist Tomogr 1991; 15:953–958.

12. Hoffmann U, Globits S, Schima W, Loewe C, Puig S, Oberhuber G, et al. Usefulness of magnetic resonance imaging of cardiac and paracardiac masses. Am J Cardiol. 2003; 92: 890–895.

13. Burke A, Virmani R. Tumors of the heart and great vessels. In: Atlas of tumor pathology. 3rd series, fasc 16. Washington, DC: Armed Forces Institute of Pathology, 1996

14. Tazelaar HD, Locke TJ, McGregor CG. Pathology of surgically excised primary cardiac tumors. Mayo Clin Proc 1992; 67:957–965.

15. Pons Lladó GJ, Ribas Garau M, Ortiz Tudanca J, Bethencourt A, Barril Baixeras R, Bonnín Gubianas JO. Heart angiosarcoma: heart magnetic resonance diagnosis. Rev Esp Cardiol 2000; 53: 1001–1004.

16. Montiel J, Ruyra X, Carreras F, Caralps JM, Aris A, Padro JM. A report of a rare case of primary angiosarcoma of left atrium and a review of the literature. Rev Esp Cardiol 1994; 47: 768–770.

17. Donatelli F, Pocar M, Moneta A, Mariani MA, Pelenghi S, Triggiani M, Santoro F, Grossi A. Primary cardiac malignancy presenting as left atrial myxoma. Clinical and surgical considerations. Minerva Chir 1996; 51: 585–588.

18. Hanson EC, Gill CC, Razavi M, Loop FD. The surgical treatment of atrial myxomas. Clinical experience and late results in 33 patients. J Thorac Cardiovasc Surg 1985; 89:298–303.

19. Grebenc ML, Rosado de Christenson ML, Green CE, Burke AP, Galvin JR. Cardiac myxoma: imaging features in 83 patients. Radiographics 2002; 22:673–89.

20. de Roos A, Weijers E, van Duinen S, van der Wall EE. Calcified right atrial myxoma demostrated by magn.etic resonance imaging. Chest 1989; 95:478–9

21. Masui T, Takahashi M, Miura K, Naito M, Tawahara K. Cardiac myxoma:identification of intratumoral hemorrage and calcification on MR images. Am J Roentgenol 1995; 164:850–2.

22. Matsuoka H, Hamada M, Honda T, Kawakami H, Abe M, Shigematsu Y, Sumimoto T, Hiwada K. Morphologic and histologic characterization of cardiac myxomas by magnetic resonance imaging. Angiology 1996;47:693–8.

23. Burke AP, Rosado-de-Christenson M, Templeton PA, Virmani R. Cardiac fibroma: clinicopathologic correlates and surgical treatment. J Thorac Cardiovasc Surg 1994; 108: 862–870.

24. Funari M, Fujita N, Peck WW, Higgins CB. Cardiac tumors: assessment with Gd-DTPA enhanced MR imaging. J Comput Asist Tomogr 1991; 15:953–8.

25. Hananouchi GI, Goff WB 2d. Cardiac lipoma: six-year follow-up with CMR characteristics, and a review of the literature. Magn Reson Imaging 1990;8(6):825–8.

26. White CS. MR evaluation of the pericardium and cardiac malignancies. Magn Reson Imaging Clin N Am 1996; 4: 237–251.

27. Reynen K. Frequency of primary tumors of the heart. Am J Cardiol 1996;77:107

28. Kapoor A: Clinical manifestations of neoplasia of the heart. In: Kapoor A, ed. Cancer of the Heart. New York: Springer-Verlag; 1986.

29. Abraham KP, Reddy V, Gattuso P. Neoplasms metastatic to the heart: review of 3314 consecutive autopsies. Am J Cardiovasc Pathol 1990; 3:195–198.

30. Tesoro-Tess JD, Biasi S, Balzarini L, Ceglia E, Matarazzo C, Piotti P, et al. Heart involvement in lymphomas. The value of magnetic resonance imaging and two-dimensional echocardiography at disease presentation. Cancer 1993; 72: 2484–2490.

31. Gibbs P, Cebon JS, Calafiore P, Robinson WA. Cardiac metastases from malignant melanoma. Cancer 1999; 85:78–84.

32. Messner G, Harting MT, Russo P, Gregoric ID, Mukhopadhyay M, Flamm SD, et al. Surgical management of metastatic melanoma to the ventricle. Tex Heart Inst J 2003; 30: 218–220.

33. Gomes AS, Lois JF, Child JS. Cardiac tumors and thrombus: evaluation with MR imaging. Am J Radiol 1987; 149:895.

34. Mohiaddin RH ed. Introduction to cardiovascular magnetic resonance. Current Medical Literature. London 2002:54.

35. Higgins CB, Caputo GR. Role of MR imaging in acquired and congenital cardiovascular disease. Am J Roentgenol 1993; 161:13–22.

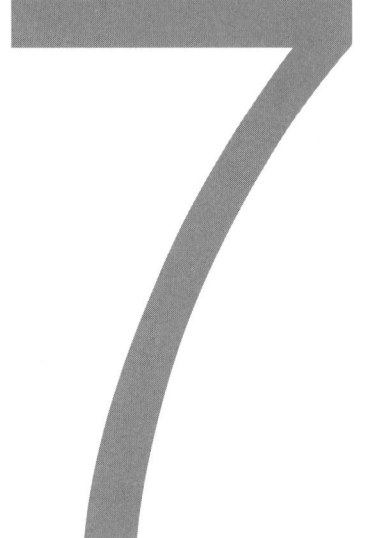

Diseases of the Pericardium

GUILLEM PONS-LLADÓ

The study of pericardial diseases is generally carried out by means of echocardiography, which is still the technique of choice in detecting effusion and diagnosing tamponade[1]. Widely available, easy to operate, and inexpensive, ultrasound are very useful in these situations. There are relevant aspects in the field of pericardial diseases, however, where echocardiography is limited, as the estimation of pericardial thickness, the detection of localized effusion, the characterization of pericardial fluid and, particularly, the study of those processes that extend beyond the limits of the heart itself.

Computed tomography (CT) and CMR, with their capacity to provide information on these aspects, have thus a definite role in the study of pericardium[2], the main advantage of CT over CMR being its ability to detect even small amounts of calcium, a determinant finding in some chronic pericardial conditions.

7.1 The Normal Pericardium

In T1w spin-echo (SE) sequences the pericardium appears as a regular curved line of low signal intensity that corresponds to the visceral and parietal components of the pericardium and to the small amount of fluid (15–50 ml) that is normally present between these fibrous layers. The visualization of this signal from the pericardial complex is in fact only possible at sites where it is encased by epicardial and paracardiac adipose tissue, of high signal intensity that strongly contrasts with the low signal intensity of the pericardium, this occuring particularly at those areas close to the right atrium and right ventricle (Figure 7.1). The pericardial space is normally 1–3 mm thick[3], provided that the measurement is performed on diastolic images, since the thickness may increase slightly in systole, and that an axial plane at the level of the inferior aspect of the heart slicing tangentially the pericardium has not been chosen. Also important is to identify the superior pericardial recesses at the level of the great vessels[2], sometimes confused with abnormal processes of the arterial wall (Figure 7.2).

7.2 Acute Pericarditis

When studied by CMR[4], patients with acute idiopathic or viral pericarditis present with pericardial effusion in 23% of cases that resolves spontaneously in most of them (Figure 7.3). In the rest of patients, in whom, in the absence of effusion, pericardial thickness can be measured, it appears slightly increased, probably as a result of the inflammatory process, this also receding after the acute phase (Figure 7.4). The mild degree of increased thickness, however, does not allow this finding to be used as an accurate sign for the diagnosis of acute pericarditis. Thus, there is no indication for a CMR study in every patient with suspected or confirmed acute pericarditis, although the technique can be useful for follow-up studies in prolonged or recurrent cases.

7.3 Pericardial Effusion

Although echocardiography is highly sensitive for the detection of pericardial effusion, the wide field of vision of CMR gives a much more detailed information on the extension and distribution of fluid. Pericardial effusion presents at CMR as an enlarged pericardial space which is generally not uniformly distributed, but, due to gravity, it tends to accumulate at the most inferior parts of the pericardial sac, as the posterior aspect or the portions adjacent to the right atrium[5] (Figure 7.5). It is known that a space larger than 5 mm between the anterior right ventricle and the parietal pericardium just beneath the anterior chest wall is indicative of a moderate degree of effusion[5]. Nevertheless, experimental studies have shown[6] that although the technique detects the presence of an infusion of pericardiac fluid of 5 ml, there is a considerable overlap of the dimensions of the effusion when the quantity of injected fluids oscillates between 40 and 120 ml, volumes which, in practical terms, would represent degrees of moderate and important effusion, respectively. It is, however, in the presence of loculated effusion where CMR shows its advantages over other techniques, thanks to the large field of view that it allows (Figure 7.6)

The ability of CMR to characterize fluid contents is useful for estimating the type of pericardiac effusion: in the most frequent type form, where the effusion consists of free serofibrinous fluid, signal intensity is typically low on T1w SE sequences and very high on gradient-echo (GRE) images (Figure 7.7), while in cine sequences a change in the shape of the pericardial space is seen during the cardiac cycle (Cine loops 7.1 and 7.2 on CD). In the case of exudates, intensity signal is intermediate on both T1w SE and GRE sequences (Figure 7.8), while in hematic effusions high signal intensity is seen on T1w SE sequences (Figure 7.9), at least in acute or subacute cases[2].

A potential cause of confusion with a pericardial effusion is the presence of an excessive amount of epicardial or paracardiac fat, not always easy to distiguish from an effusion in echocardiographic studies. The characteristic high signal intensity of adipose tissue on T1w SE sequences, togheter with the ability to detect the signal corresponding to the pericardium, make CMR an optimal technique to rule out pericardial effusion in these cases (Figure 7.10).

7.4 Constrictive Pericarditis

The diagnosis of pericardial constriction is based on the documentation of the presence of an abnormal pericardium, wich is sometimes easily done by means of a plain chest X-ray, when there is extensive pericardial calcification, although not rarely another imaging technique is required. While CT is often the first choice[1], mainly due to its ability to detect even small amount of calcium, CMR is also a reliable technique in the study of pericardial constriction.

An abnormal thickening of the pericardium, in a patient with clinical data suggestive of constriction, is virtually diagnostic, helping to exclude myocardial restriction. On T1w SE sequences, an increase in the width of the low intensity signal of the pericardium can be observed, indicating the presence of an abnormally thickened fibrous pericardial component in the pericardium. As an enlarged pericardial space with low signal intensity on SE images may also be seen in simple pericardial effusion,

FIGURE 7.1

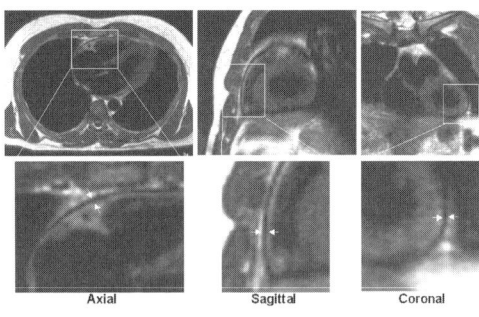

Axial   Sagittal   Coronal

FIGURE 7.2

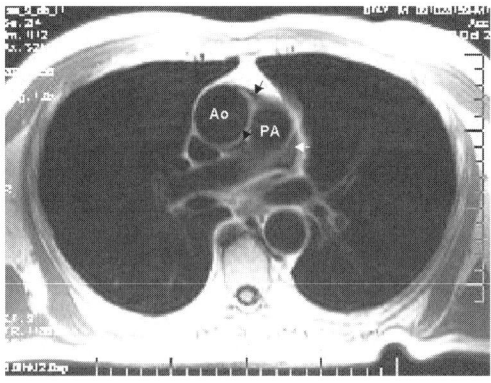

FIGURE 7.3

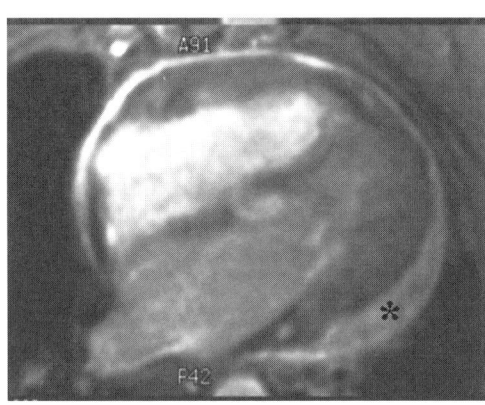

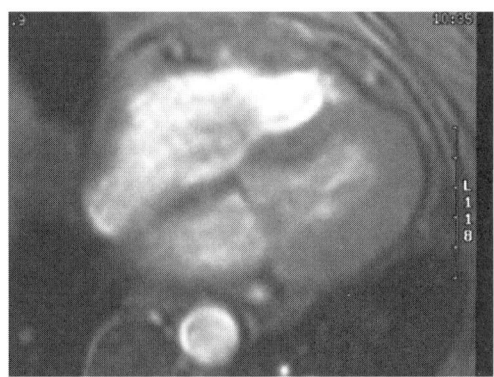

FIGURE 7.4

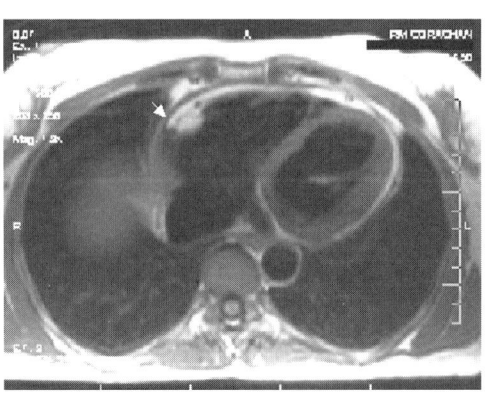

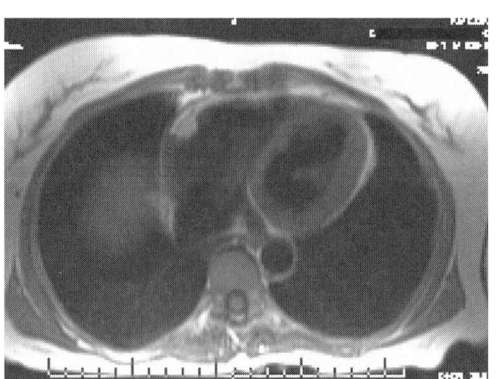

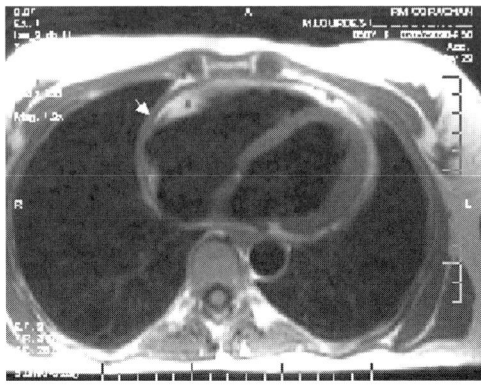

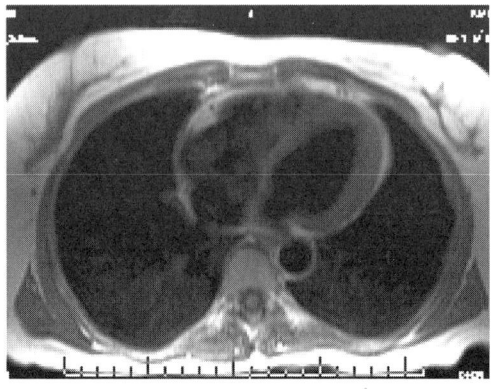

FIGURE 7.5

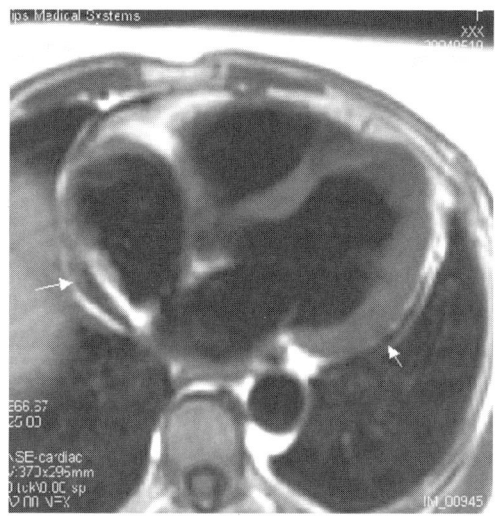 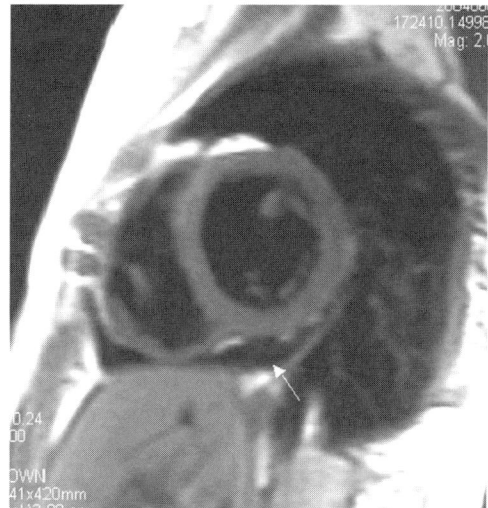

FIGURE 7.6

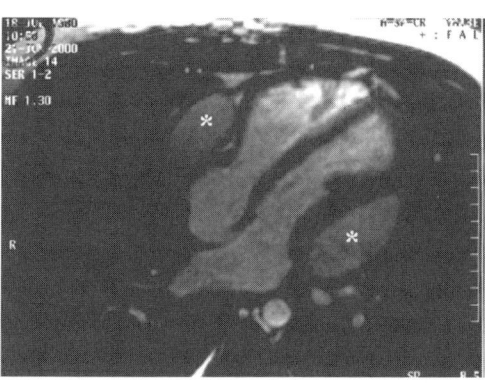

F. 7.1. Appearance of the normal pericardium on axial, sagittal and coronal thoracic T1w SE images. Observe that the pericardium is only visualized at those areas (enlarged at the bottom) where the presence of fat produces a high signal intensity allowing the much lower intense pericardial signal to be clearly delineated.

F. 7.2. Normal axial plane on T1w SE at the level of the ascending aorta (Ao) and the pulmonary artery (PA), where the anterior and posterior aortic recesses (black arrows) are seen, as well as the left pulmonic recess (white arrow).

F. 7.3. Axial plane in GRE at the ventricular level in a patient during (left panel) and months after (right panel) an apparently uncomplicated episode of acute pericarditis. Observe the presence of pericardial effusion the acute phase (asterisk) and its disappearance at follow-up.

F. 7.4. Axial T1w SE images showing, at left, a mildly increased pericardial thickness (arrows) during the acute phase of an episode of pericarditis. The images at right correspond to the same location than those at left, and were obtained from the same patients some months after clinical recovery: the pericardial thickness is now within normal limits.

F. 7.5. Axial (left panel) and short-axis (right) planes on T1w SE showing pericardial effusion with the fluid mainly occupying the inferior and posterior aspects of the pericardial sac.

F. 7.6. Horizontal longitudinal plane on a GRE sequence showing a loculated pericardial effusion with a peculiar distribution of fluid, surrounding the atrioventricular plane of the heart (asterisks).

FIGURE 7.7

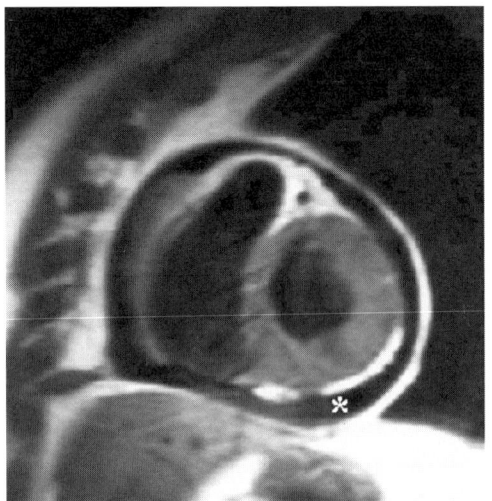
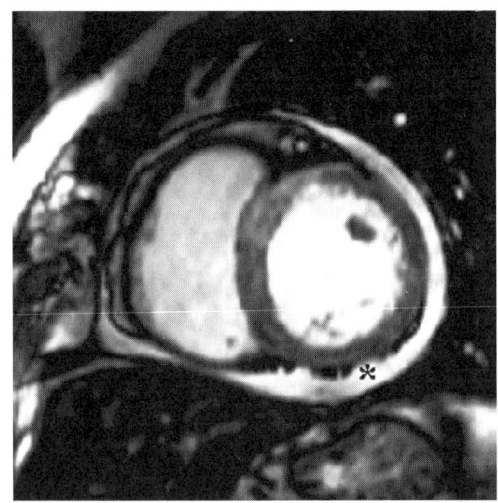

FIGURE 7.8

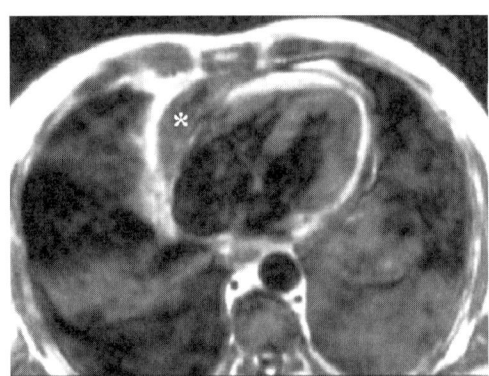
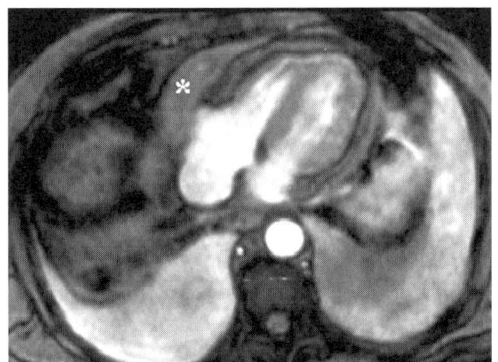

FIGURE 7.9

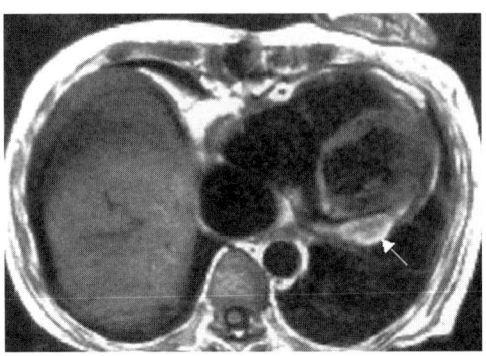
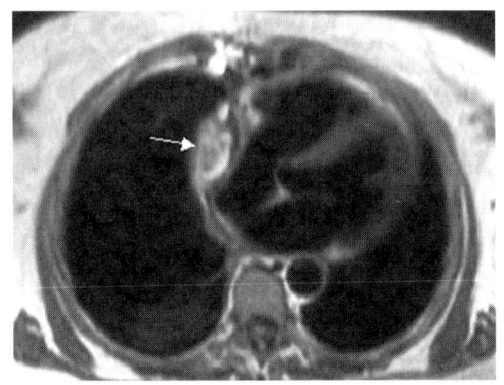

FIGURE 7.10

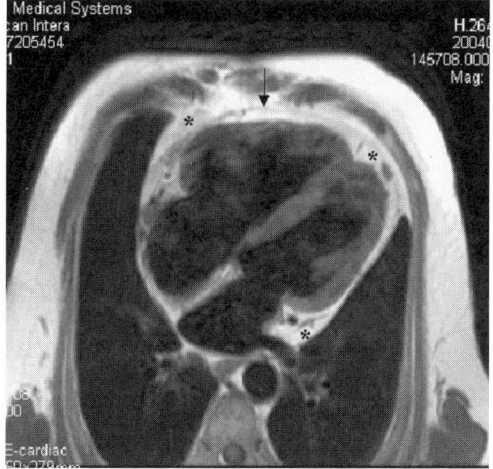

F. 7.7.   T1w SE (left panel) and GRE (right) images from the same patient, showing the signal intensity of a serous pericardial effusion (asterisks): low on SE and high on GRE.

F. 7.8.   Axial planes on T1w SE (left panel) and GRE (right) from the same patient, showing pericardial effusion (asterisks) with intermediate signal intensity on both sequences, corresponding to a case of exudative effusion.

F. 7.9.   Axial planes on T1w SE in two cases of loculated pericardial hematoma (asterisks), both after heart surgery. Note the high signal intensity of the effusion, indicating its hematic contents.

F. 7.10. Axial T1w SE image in a patient with profuse amounts of epicardial and paracardiac fat (asteriks). Note the thin line of the normal pericardium (arrow) inside the adipose tissue.

GRE sequences are also helpful, as the presence of fluid is detected here by an increase in signal, on contrast with pericardial thickening without effusion (Figure 7.11). Pericardial thickening in constrictive pericarditis is typically diffuse, although not uniform. Moreover, it it can be only detected by CMR at those areas where the presence of epicardial fat provides a natural contrast allowing the measurement of the pericardial thickness. Once confirmed that a pericardial effusion is absent, a thickness over 4 mm, in a patient with clinical data consistent with constriction has a high diagnostic accuracy for the diagnosis[7].

Unfortunately, the presence of pericardial calcification, wich is a useful diagnostic sign of constriction, does not produce but a nonspecific signal absence in most CMR sequences, although there are other indirect findings of constriction, as is the presence of an abnormal early diastolic flattening of the interventricular septum (Figure 7.12, and Cine loop 7.3 on CD), as a result of the increased hemodynamic dependence of both ventricles in constriction[8], a narrowed tubular-shaped right ventricle (Figure 7.13), or a dilated vena cava (Figure 7.14), as an expression of congestive heart failure.

As indirect signs, however, these findings can be modified by an eventual medical treatment, and, therefore, have limited diagnostic value[7]. The important point is still the assessment of pericardial thickness, a finding that, even when appropriately determined by CMR, must be evaluated in the clinical context of the patient. Thus, on one side, the mere detection of an increased pericardial thickness does not mean constriction[9] (Figure 7.15), as it can be seen in situations such as those following cardiac surgery[10] or during the acute phase of a simple pericarditis[4] (Figure 7.4). On the other hand, it is known that in between 10%[7] and 20%[5] of the cases of pericardial constriction no significantly increased thickness of the pericardium is noted by CMR, a finding that has been also reported after histopathological studies in a similar proportion of patients with surgically proven pericardial constriction[11].

7.5 Congenital Pericardial Diseases

An infrequent abnormality, the *congenital absence of the pericardium* is frequently partial and affects the left portion of the pericardium, the patients being generally asymptomatic. It is usually detected in the form of an apparent cardiomegaly at chest X-rays, due in fact to an abnormal displacement of the heart, CMR being always useful for the diagnosis[12]. The simple apparent lack of signal corresponding to the pericardium in CMR images has no diagnostic value, since, as stated previously, it is frequently not visualized in its whole extension (Figure 7.1). The study of the relationships of cardiovascular mediastinal structures is useful for the diagnosis, as it shows that, although the cardiac chambers are markedly displaced, they are otherwise not

FIGURE 7.11

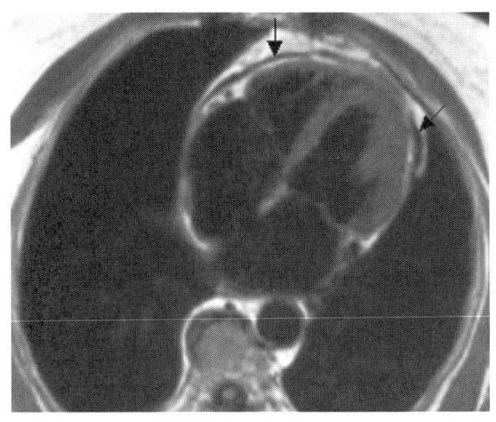
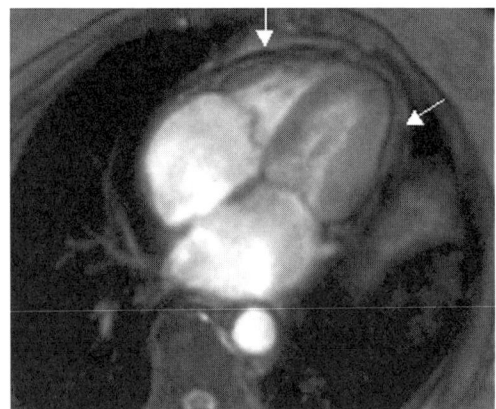

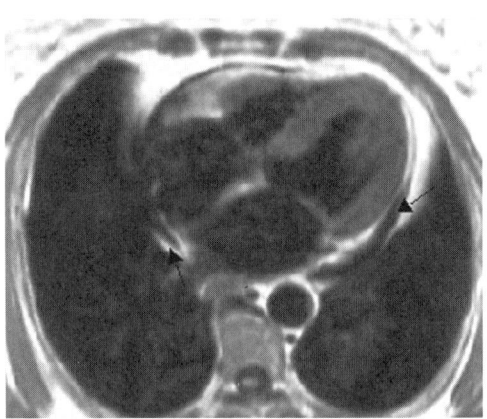
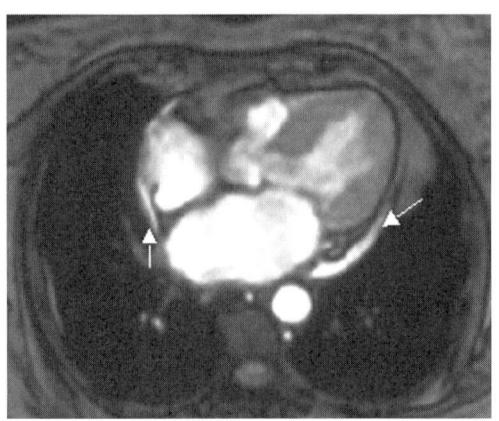

FIGURE 7.12

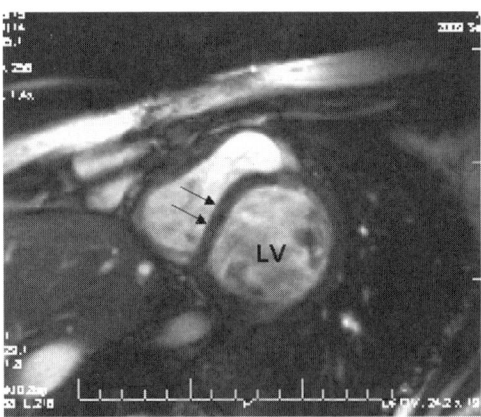

FIGURE 7.13

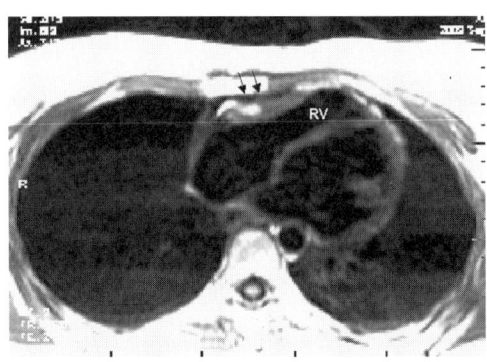

F. 7.11. Top left panel: T1w SE axial plane from a patient with constrictive pericarditis, showing an increased pericardial space with low intensity signal (black arrows); Top right: GRE image on the same patient: no high intensity signal is noted at the pericardial level (white arrows); Bottom left: T1w SE axial plane in a case of mild pericardial effusion, showing increased pericardial space, also with low-intensity signal (black arrows); Bottom right: the corresponding GRE image, in this case showing high signal intensity (white arrows) indicating the presence of pericardial fluid. Compare with the images at top, and observe the different distribution of the enlargement of the pericardial space, wich distributes at the lowermost areas of the pericardial sac in the case of effusion (bottom).

FIGURE 7.14

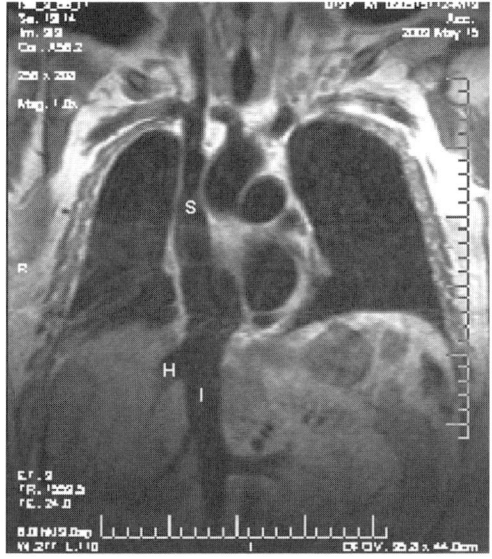 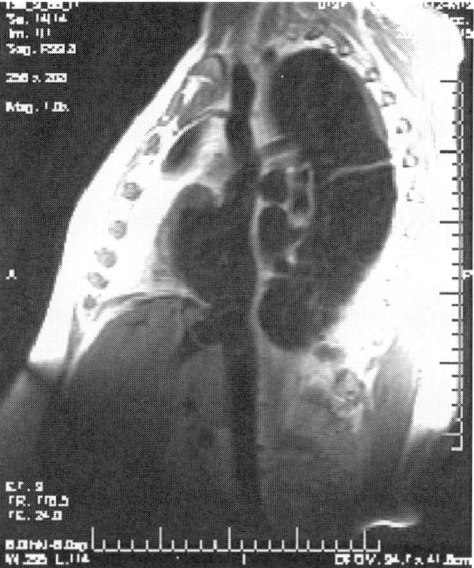

FIGURE 7.15

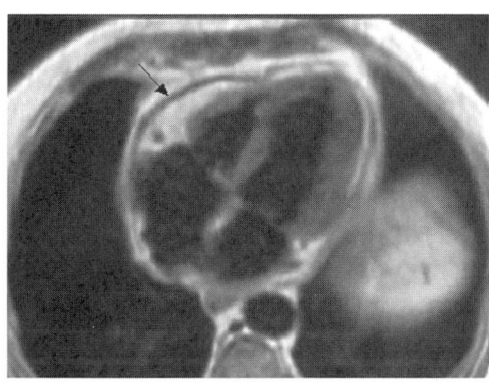 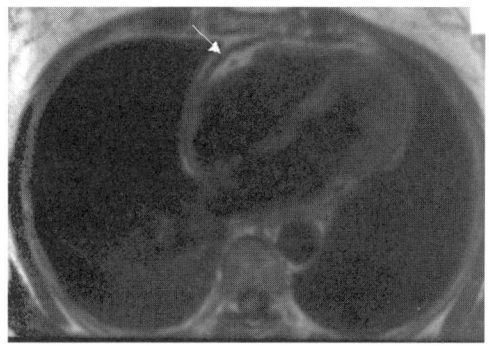

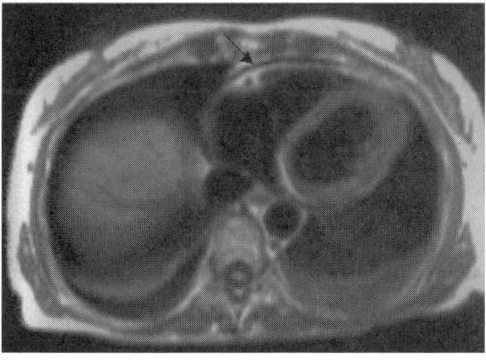 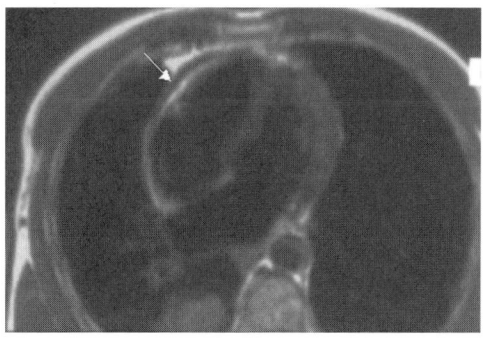

F. 7.12. Early diastolic (left panel) and end-systolic (right) frames from a cine sequence on a short-axis level of the heart, showing a flattening of the interventricular septum (arrows), that looses its concave shape towards the left ventricle (LV).

F. 7.13. Tubular shaped narrowing of the right ventricle (RV) in a patient with a localized anterior constrictive pericarditis (arrows).

F. 7.14. Coronal (left panel) and sagittal (right) thoracic planes showing dilatation of the superior (S) and inferior (I) vena cava and, also, of the hepatic vein (H),in a patient with constrictive pericarditis.

F. 7.15. Axial T1w SE images at the level of the ventricles in four different cases: the two patients on the left exhibit pericardial thickening (black arrows) but were free of clinical symptoms of constriction; the two on the right did actually suffer from constrictive pericarditis that required surgery, despite of similar degrees of pericardial thickening at CMR (white arrows).

dilated. Also, and importantly, the mediastinal extrapericardial structures, such as the great vessels, maintain their normal position despite of some distortion at the root of the arteries, wich is the cause of an useful finding, as is the presence of a "tongue" of lung tissue interposing between the main pulmonary artery and aorta[12] (Figure 7.16). The importance of detecting the presence of a congenital absence of the pericardium is the potential risk of strangulation of cardiac structures, which require surgical treatment, and that up to 30% of cases are associated with other intracardiac congenital malformations[13].

The *pericardial cyst* is a benign lesion that originates during embryonic development of the pericardium and which is frequently asymptomatic. It is usually detected after a chest X-ray shows an abnormal cardiac shape, often located in the right anterior cardiophrenic region. Its clear fluid content and sharp definition of its edges cause the CMR images to be always demonstrative, appearing as a well delineated mass with typical cystic features[14]: round or ovoid shape, with an homogeneously low or intermediate signal intensity on T1w SE sequences, which increases in T2w images (Figure 7.17).

FIGURE 7.16

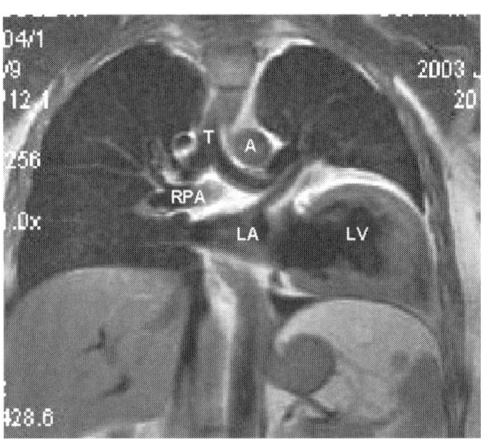 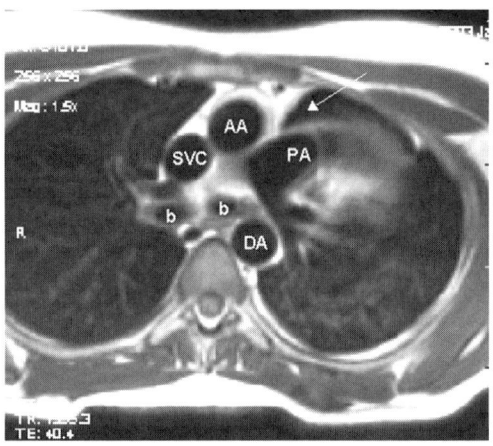

FIGURE 7.17

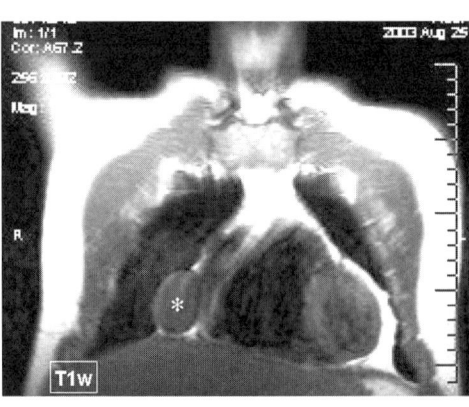 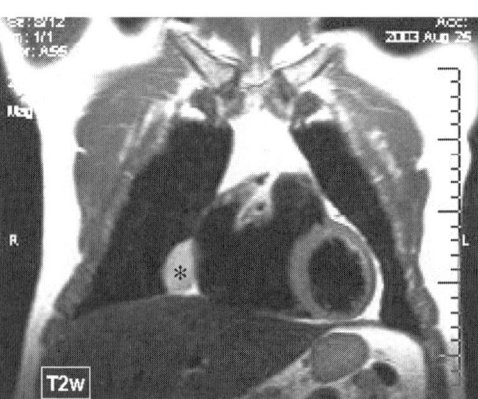

F. 7.16. Coronal (left panel) and axial (right) planes on T1w SE on a patient with congenital absence of the left pericardium. Note the marked leftward displacement of the heart with a normal position of the mediastinal structures (left), and the interposition of a "tongue" of lung tissue (arrow, on the right panel) between the great arteries. A: aortic arch; AA: ascending aorta; b: bronchi; DA: descending aorta; LA: left atrium; LV: left ventricle; PA: pulmonary artery (main trunk); RPA: right pulmonary artery; SVC: superior vena cava; T: trachea.

F. 7.17. Coronal T1w SE (left panel) and T2w SE (right) in a patient with a congenital pericardial cyst located at the right cardiophrenic angle. Note the intermediate signal intensity of the cyst on the T1w sequence (white asterisk), that appears highly intense on the T2w image (black asterisk).

References

1. Breen JF. Imaging of the pericardium. J Thorac Imaging. 2001; 16: 47–54.

2. Wang ZJ, Reddy GP, Gotway MB, Yeh BM, Hetts SW, Higgins CB. CT and MR imaging of pericardial disease. Radiographics 2003; 23: S167-S180.

3. Sechtem U, Tscholakoff D, Higgins CB. MRI of the normal pericardium. Am J Roentgenol 1986; 147: 239–244.

4. Pons-Lladó G, Carreras F. Borrás X, Palmer J, Llauger J, Jiménez-Borreguero LJ, et al. MRI in acute pericarditis. Preliminary results of a Spanish Collaborative Study (abstr.). J Cardiovasc Magn Reson 1999; 4: 379.

5. Sechtem U, Tscholakoff D, Higgins CB. MRI of the abnormal pericardium. Am J Roentgenol 1986; 147: 245–252.

6. Rokey R, Vick III GW, Bolli R, Lewandowski ED. Assessment of experimental pericardial effusion using nuclear magnetic resonance imaging techniques. Am Heart J 1991; 121: 1161–1169.

7. Masui T, Finck S, Higgins CB. Constrictive pericarditis and restrictive cardiomyopathy: evaluation with MR imaging. Radiology 1992; 182: 369–373.

8. Giorgi B, Mollet NR, Dymarkowski S, Rademakers FE, Bogaert J. Clinically suspected constrictive pericarditis: MR imaging assessment of ventricular septal motion and configuration in patients and healthy subjects. Radiology 2003; 228: 417–424.

9. Axel L. Assessment of pericardial disease by magnetic resonance and computed tomography. J Magn Reson Imaging 2004; 19: 816–826.

10. Duvernoy O, Malm T, Thuomas KA, Larsson SG, Hansson HE. CT and MR evaluation of pericardial and retrosternal adhesions after cardiac surgery. J Comput Assist Tomogr 1991; 15: 555–560.

11. Talreja DR, Edwards WD, Danielson GK, Schaff HV, Tajik AJ, Tazelaar HD, et al. Constrictive pericarditis in 26 patients with histologically normal pericardial thickness. Circulation. 2003; 108: 1852–1857.

12. Gatzoulis MA, Munk MD, Merchant N, Van Arsdell GS, McCrindle BW, Webb GD. Isolated congenital absence of the pericardium: clinical presentation, diagnosis, and management. Ann Thorac Surg 2000; 69:1209–1215.

13. White CS. MR evaluation of the pericardium and cardiac malignancies. Magn Reson Imaging Clin N Am 1996; 4: 237–252.

14. Murayama S, Murakami J, Watanabe H, Sakai S, Hinaga S, Soeda H, et al. Signal intensity characteristics of mediastinal cystic masses on T1 weighted MRI. J Comput Assist Tomogr 1995; 19: 188–191.

Congenital Heart Disease

8

MAITE SUBIRANA
XAVIER BORRÁS

Cardiovascular magnetic resonance (CMR) is an extremely useful tool to study congenital heart disease, as it has the main advantages of both echocardiography and conventional angiography[1, 2, 3, 4, 5, 6]. Like ultrasound, CMR is a noninvasive technique providing accurate morphological information on the heart and, as angiography, it allows the study of extracardiac vascular structures. This latter characteristic is very important, because it permits to evaluate the ventriculo-arterial connections, the position and relationship between the great arteries and the drainage of the systemic and pulmonary veins[7]. An additional advantage of CMR that should be noted is its excellent image quality in the majority of patients, including adults[8] and those who have been submitted to surgical cardiac correction, as it does not require a particular window to obtain adequate images[9], neither it has limitations in the orientation of views, and it can produce images in any desired plane of the heart[10].

8.1 Segmental Study of Congenital Heart Disease

In the study of congenital anomalies of the heart and the great vessels the description of the position and morphology of cardiovascular structures as well as the existing connections between them is very important. This is known as segmental analysis of the heart. The diagnosis of cardiac malpositions and of the *situs* can be approached using radiology, electrocardiography or echocardiography, but the study of venous drainage, atrioventricular and ventriculoarterial connections as well as the relative position of the different cardiac segments, especially in the case of complex cardiac anomalies, is more reliably performed by CMR.

8.2 Study of Atria and Venous connections

The first step consists in the assessment of the position and orientation of the heart within the thoracic cavity (levocardia, dextrocardia or mesocardia) (Figure 8.1). The following step is the determination of the atrial *situs*. The morphologically right atrium is normally located anteriorly and to the right. It is characterized by a triangular-shaped atrial appendage with a wide connection to the rest of the atrium. The morphologically left atrium has smoother walls and an appendage that is narrower and finger-like shaped. The situation where a morphologically right atrium is situated to the right of a morphologically left atrium (normal position) is known as atrial *situs solitus* (Figure 8.2). When the morphologically left atrium is placed anterior and to the right of a morphologically right atrium, it is known as atrial *situs inversus*. When both atria have similar morphology (both right or both left), it is known as atrial *isomerism* (right or left respectively) and the *situs* is called *situs ambiguus*. CMR has shown a high capacity to determine the atrial and thoracic *situs*, since segmental anatomy is optimally displayed in transverse and coronal planes. By means of spin-echo (SE) techniques it is possible to identify the morphologically left and right atrium as well as the left and the right main bronchi, which is of great help, because usually there is a spatial concordance between those structures, atrium and bronchi. Likewise, as provided its wide field of view, CMR also allows the analysis of the abdominal *situs*,[11] which is generally concordant with the atrial and thoracic *situs*. In case of discordance between the atrial and the visceral *situs*, a diagnosis of *situs ambiguus* can be advanced; it is almost always associated with the asplenia (right atrial isomerism) or polysplenia (left atrial isomerism) syndromes.

Systemic venous blood return can help in assessing the atrial *situs*. In *situs solitus*, the inferior vena cava is located to the right of the vertebral column and drains into a morphologically right atrium, placed on the right. In *situs inversus*, the inferior vena cava is located to the left of the vertebral column and drains into a morphologically right atrium, placed on the left. In cases of *situs ambiguus,* associated with a syndrome of polysplenia, the suprahepatic veins usually drain directly into the atrium. The syndrome is characterized by two morphologically left atria, two long main bronchi (morphologically left), a central liver, multiple spleens and interruption of the inferior vena cava with continuation of the abdominal venous blood return through the system of the azygos or hemiazygos veins. In *situs ambiguus* associated with a syndrome of asplenia, the two atrial cavities are morphologically right, the two main bronchi are short (morphologically right), the liver is placed in the middle of the abdominal cavity, there is not spleen and the inferior vena cava and the abdominal aorta are usually situated on the same side of the vertebral column with the vein in an antero-lateral position. By using axial, coronal and sagittal slices, the position, course and flow of the inferior vena cava can be observed by CMR. It is a very useful technique not only for identifying situs but also for the study of the anomalies of systemic venous return. In case of interruption of the inferior vena cava, the level of interruption and the venous abdominal return through the azygos and hemiazygos veins can be detected, especially using coronal planes. Likewise, a direct drainage of suprahepatic veins into the atrium can be easily displayed (Figure 8.3).

The superior vena cava usually drains into a morphologically right atrium. A dilated superior vena cava suggests either an anomaly causing systemic venous hypertension, or an obstruction of the drainage of this vein. (Figure 8.4).

A frequent abnormality of the systemic venous return is a persistent left superior vena cava, that generally drains into a dilated coronary sinus. It may be easily diagnosed by CMR (Figure 8.5).

The coronary sinus is seen in axial planes behind the morphologically left atrium. As has been noted previously, a dilated coronary sinus suggests as a first diagnostic option a persistent left superior vena cava; however, it may be seen in cases of anomalous drainage of the pulmonary veins or arteriovenous fistula draining into it.

The four pulmonary veins drain into the left atrium through its posterior wall and can be easily visualized by using both the SE and the gradient-echo (GRE) CMR techniques. There are different types of anomalies of the pulmonary venous return, depending on the number of pulmonary veins involved (partial or total anomalous pulmonary venous connection) and on the draining structure (into the

FIGURE 8.1

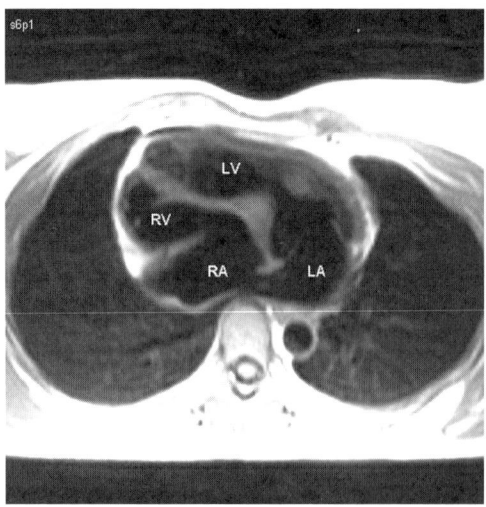

FIGURE 8.2

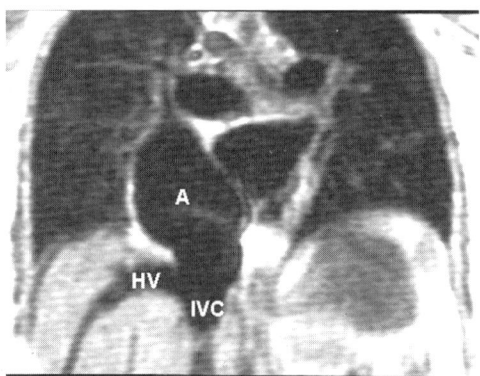 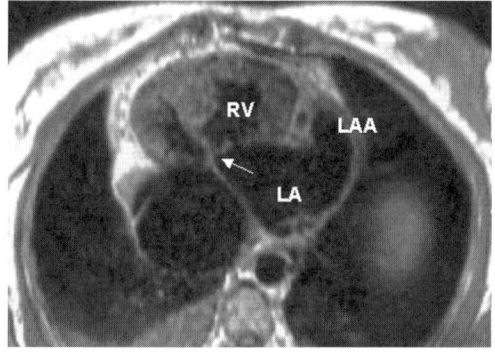

FIGURE 8.3

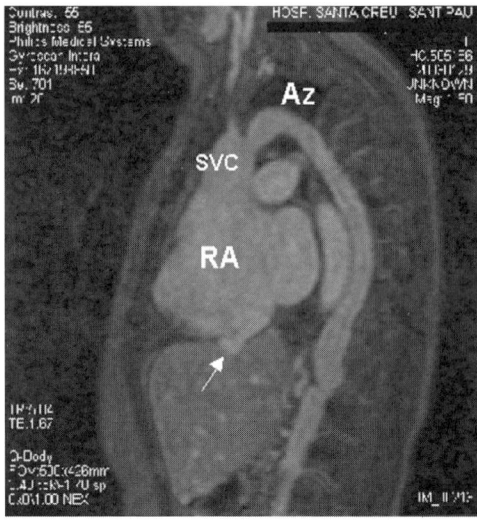 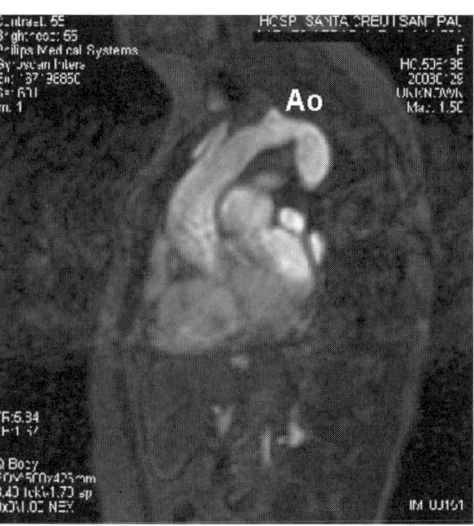

F. 8.1.   Axial "black-blood" Fast SE showing isolated dextrocardia: the heart is placed on the right hemithorax. LA: left atrium; LV: left ventricle; RA: right atrium; RV: right ventricle.

F. 8.2.   Clues for the diagnosis of *situs* and the identification of cardiac chambers. Left panel: coronal T1wSE image showing (1) an inferior vena cava (IVC) and an hepatic vein (HV) situated on the right, draining into an atrium (A) placed on the right, this suggesting the diagnosis of *situs solitus*. Right panel: Axial plane from the same patient showing: (2) a heart placed on the right side of the chest (dextrocardia) with the apex directed toward the right (dextroversion); (3) a morphologically left atrial appendage (LAA) (finger-like shape) situated on the left, this identifying the left atrium (LA); (4) a septal insertion of the left atrioventricular valve closer to the the apex (arrow) than the right one, this identifying the former as the tricuspid valve and, thus, the ventricle connected to it as morphologically right (RV). The patient can be considered as suffering from a complex congenital heart disease with: dextrocardia, dextroversion, *situs solitus* and atrioventricular discordance.

FIGURE 8.4

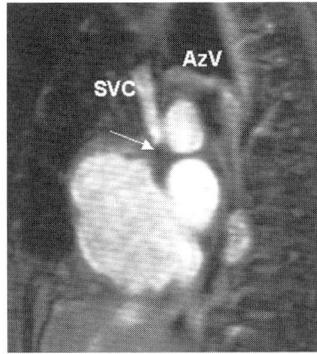 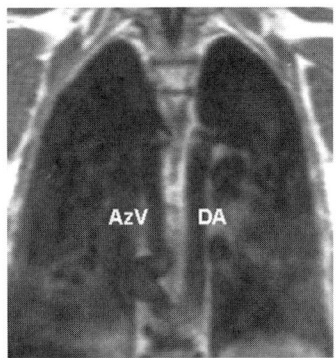 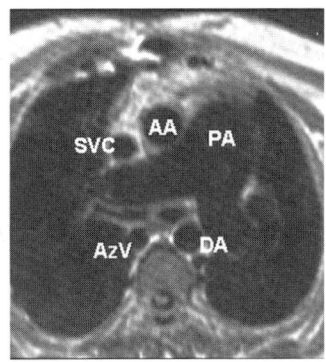

FIGURE 8.5

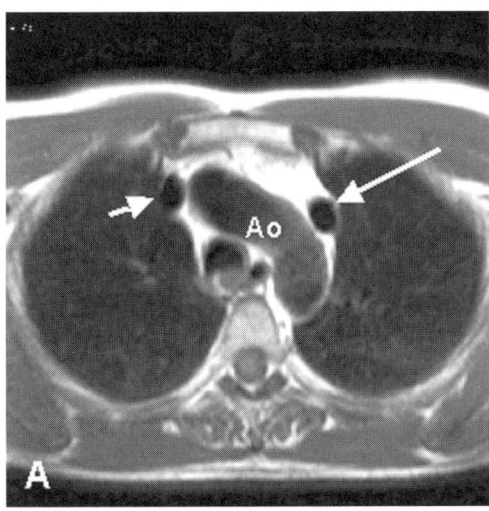 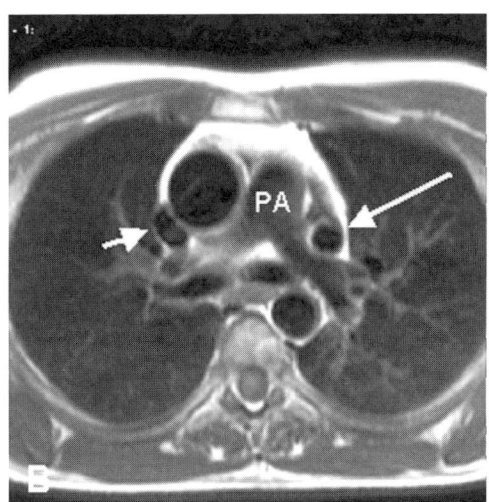

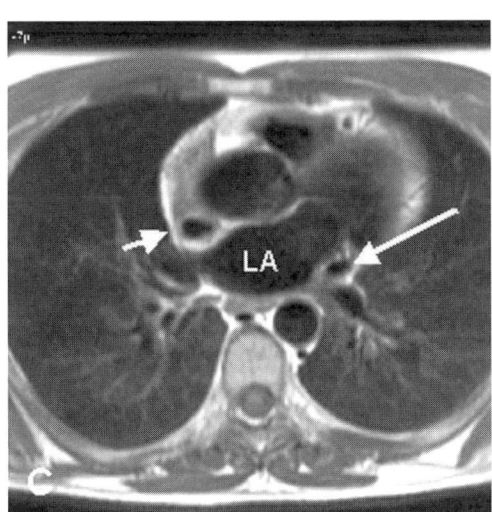 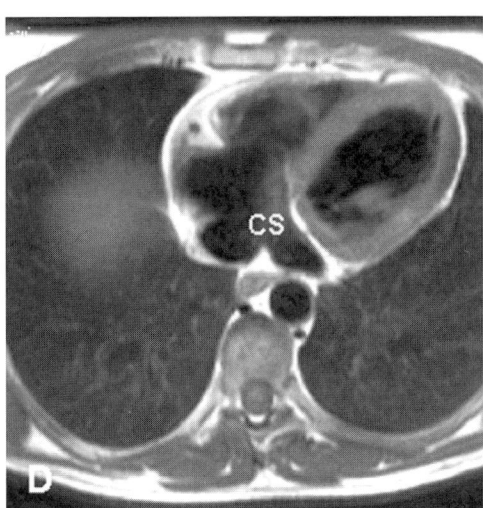

F. 8.3. Sagittal planes from the stack of an MR angiography in a case of congenital absence of inferior vena cava showing, at left, a compensatory enlargement of the azygos vein (Az) draining into the superior vena cava (SVC); the arrow points to a collector of the hepatic veins directly connected to the right atrium (RA). The right panel corresponds to a plane parallel to the one on the left showing the thoracic aorta (Ao).

F. 8.4. Obstruction of the superior vena cava (SVC) after a surgical closure of a *sinus venosus* atrial septal defect. Left panel: sagittal GRE image showing the interruption of the SVC at level of the drainage into the atrium (arrow) and a collateral circulation through the azygos vein (AzV). Middle panel: coronal T1w SE plane showing the enlarged AzV, with a diameter equivalent to that of the descending aorta (DA). Right panel: axial T1w SE plane displaying the enlarged AzV on a crossectional plane. AA: ascending aorta; PA: pulmonary artery.

F. 8.5. Axial "black-blood" Fast SE planes on descending order from A to D, showing a persistent left superior vena cava (long arrow) that courses laterally to the aortic arch (Ao), the pulmonary artery (PA) and the left atrium (LA), and drains into a dilated coronary sinus (CS); a normal right superior vena cava (short arrow) coexists, in this case.

FIGURE 8.6

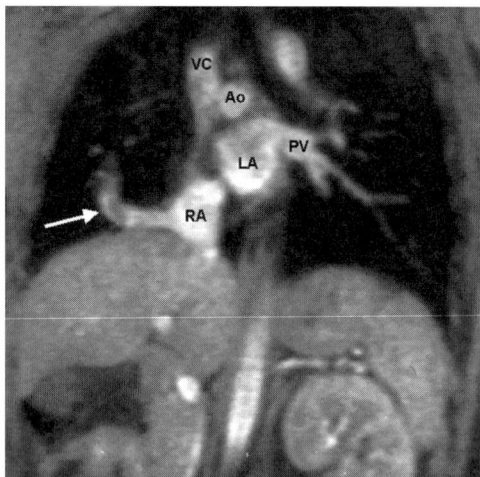

F. 8.6. Coronal GRE section showing an anomalous right pulmonary venous drainage (arrow) into the right atrium (RA) in a patient with a scimitar's syndrome; left pulmonary vein (PV) is seen draining into the left atrium (LA). Ao: aorta; VC: superior vena cava.

into intracardiac structures (coronary sinus, right atrium) or into extracardiac ones (right superior vena cava, azygos vein, innominate vein, left superior vena cava), or at infradiaphragmatic level (inferior vena cava or portal system). This last situation is usually associated with an obstruction of the pulmonary venous return and as a consequence, with pulmonary venous hypertension. The wide field of view of CMR allows to visualize the complete courses of TPAVD, including pulmonary veins, pulmonary venous confluence, vertical veins, and entrance of the vertical veins, usually providing all what is needed for the diagnosis. However, as this abnormality presents with early clinical symptoms, the diagnosis is usually achieved by echocardiography, being CMR more useful in the postoperative control of these patients. It may help to detect some residual lesions or sequels requiring a further surgical intervention (5–20% of the cases)[14], as may be an obstruction of the pulmonary venous return.[15]

right atrium, into the superior vena cava, into the inferior vena cava, into the coronary sinus, etc.). CMR is much more useful than echocardiography to diagnose an anomalous pulmonary venous drainage (sensitivity: 95% versus 38%), being even superior to angiography (sensitivity: 69%).[12] Axial planes are usually enough to diagnose the anomaly, but in some cases the use of additional sagital or coronal planes may be necessary (Figure 8.6). The identification of any one of the four pulmonary veins draining into the left atrium excludes the diagnosis of a total anomalous pulmonary venous connection.

The *sinus venosus* type of atrial septal defect is frequently associated with a partial anomalous pulmonary venous drainage. The right superior pulmonary vein drains into the right atrium or the superior vena cava. In the latter case, using axial planes a defect is observed in the lateral wall of the superior vena cava, a typical image that has been described as the sign of the "broken ring."[13]

In total anomalous pulmonary venous drainage (TAPVD), the pulmonary veins usually converge in a common collector. It may drain at supradiaphragmatic level, either

8.3 Atrioventricular Connections

The ventricles may be identified on the basis of their morphology and on the anatomical characteristics of the atrioventricular valves. The right ventricle usually displays a triangular form on axial planes, with a coarse trabecular pattern and with the moderator band situated near the apex. The left ventricle presents with an elliptical form with a smoother septal surface. Another anatomic feature that is useful in identifying the cardiac chambers is the fact that the atrio-ventricular valve always belongs to the appropriate ventricle; thus, the mitral valve is always found in the morphologically left ventricle, and the tricuspid valve in the morphologically right ventricle. We can identify the tricuspid valve because it inserts in the interventricular septum closer to the apex than the mitral valve, and because it has chordal insertions into the ventricular septum. The mitral valve has chordal insertions into two papillary muscles and is a bicuspid, fish-mouth shaped valve.

Atrioventricular concordance describes the situation where the morphologically right atrium is connected to the morphologically right ventricle and the morphologically left atrium to the morphologically left ventricle. The connection is called discordant when the morphologically right atrium connects to the morphologically left ventricle and the morphologically left atrium connects to the morphologically right ventricle, independently of the spatial position of the chambers (Figure 8.2). In cases of atrial isomerism the atrioventricular connexion is known as ambiguous. There are other types of atrioventricular connexions, as when the two atria connect directly to a single ventricle (double inlet atrioventricular connection) and when only one atrium is connected to a ventricular inlet portion. In the later arrangement, the other atrioventricular connection is absent (tricuspid or mitral atresia). Because of this, a rudimentary ventricular chamber may be present, which does not receive an inlet portion. Some authors group hearts with double inlet or with absence on one atrioventricular connection together as univentricular hearts.

The type of atrioventricular connection (concordant, discordant, ambiguous, double inlet and absent right or left) should be differentiated from the mode of atrioventricular connection. The mode describes the specific morphology of the valve apparatus and may occur with any type of connection. When there are two atrioventricular connections, these may be through two patent atrioventricular valves, through a common atrioventricular valve, or through the combination of a permeable valve and an imperforate valve. At the same time an incorrect alignment of the connection may exist (valve in overriding or straddling position).

CMR is a useful technique to study the atrioventricular connections, specially by using the axial planes in SE sequences. In some cases of complex anomalies it could be necessary to use views with an oblique orientation, although planes different from the standard ones not infrequently lead to confusion in the study of congenital heart disease, where structures may be grossly distorted. One of the limitations of the technique is its suboptimal resolution in the visualization of valves as they are thin and move rapidly. Then, some valvular abnormalities, as mitral or tricuspid valve prolapse, myxoid degeneration, clefts, imperforation, etc. are better studied by echocardiography.

8.4 Ventriculoarterial Connections

When the pulmonary artery originates from a morphologically right ventricle and the aorta arises from a morphologically left ventricle (more than 50% of the sigmoid annulus arising from the ventricular chamber), the ventriculoarterial connexion is called concordant. When the morphologically left ventricle connects to the pulmonary artery and the morphologically right ventricle to the aorta, a ventriculoarterial discordance occurs, independently from the spatial position of the different chambers and/or vessels. The term "transposition" should be reserved for defining a type of relationship of the great vessels and it is important to remember that any relationship may occur with any arterial connection. In a normal anatomic pattern, the aorta is placed posterior and to the left of the pulmonary artery, and the outflow tract of the right ventricle is wrapped anteriorly around the left ventricular outflow tract and aortic root. When the aorta is situated in a position anterior to the pulmonary artery then the great vessels are in transposition, L-transposition occurring when the aorta is anterior and to the left of the pulmonary artery, and D-transposition when it is placed anterior and to the right of the pulmonary artery. Identification and position of the great arteries may be easily done by magnetic resonance. The aorta gives rise to brachiocephalic and coronary arteries, whereas the main pulmonary artery bifurcates into right and left pulmonary branches. In contrast to echocardiography, CMR has no restrictions in displaying views of the great vessels. This usually allows to identify them easily, to study their relationship and to describe the type of ventriculoarterial connection. Likewise, it permits the evaluation of the size of the aorta and the pulmonary arteries,[16] including the main and the distal pulmonary arteries, and may be specially useful in diagnosing branch pulmonary artery discontinuity and stenosis, which is very important in the evaluation of surgical possibilities.

To visualize the pulmonary artery bifurcation (the clue for its identification), CMR axial planes of the thorax are usually the most useful (Figure 8.7). They also provide information about the position of the ascending aorta, normally placed posterior and to the right of the pulmonary artery, and of the descending aorta, which under normal conditions runs along the left side of the vertebral column. Coronal planes are generally useful for the study of the ascending aorta and the aortic arch branches. Mild angulations of these planes may improve the visualization of these structures. Cine CMR technique permits to study blood flow conditions and to detect possible anomalies in it. Additionally, the velocity mapping technique can be used to measure the flow into different vascular structures.

8.5 Study of Shunts

A frequent abnormality in congenital heart disease is the presence of defects allowing communication between the systemic and the pulmonary circulation, that permit shunting of blood. Usually, the shunt is left-to-right causing an increase in pulmonary flow. The shunt can be isolated or be associated with other congenital anomalies, in which case the shunting of blood can be essential for the survival of the patient, as occurs in cases of some congenital heart anomalies ductus arteriosus dependent.

The study of shunts requires an appropriate assessment of: 1) the morphology, size and level (atrial, ventricular, great vessels, etc.) of the defect, 2) the direction and volume of the shunt, and 3) its hemodynamic overload on the heart.

The most frequent shunts can be found in the following malformations: atrial septal defect, ventricular septal defect and patent ductus arteriosus. Other shunts may be the result of an anomalous pulmonary venous drainage, an aortopulmonary window or an arteriovenous fistula. The fistula can be localized at different levels, the most frequent being the pulmonary and coronary fistulas (Figure 8.8). A special type of arteriovenous communication is the one that can be established between the aorta and the pulmonary artery in cases of an anomalous origin of the left coronary artery from the main pulmonary artery (Figure 8.9). In this anomaly, flow from the right coronary artery may drain into the pulmonary trunk through collateral arteries

that connect both coronary arteries (right and left). If the shunt is important, it can cause myocardial ischemia due to a stealing phenomenon.

CMR is a valuable tool for volume quantification of cardiovascular shunts. Two methods are avalaible: the volumetric technique and the flow quantification technique. The first approach is based on the calculation of end-diastolic and end-systolic right and left ventricular volumes on series of short-axis planes of the ventricles on GRE cine sequences (see Chapter 2). The shunt volume is calculated as the difference between right and left ventricular absolute stroke volumes. This method can not be used for quantifying the shunt volume in ventricular septal defects, and may be mistaken in cases of associated aortic and/or pulmonary regurgitation. The second method is based on phase-velocity cine magnetic resonance imaging. The blood flow is measured in the main pulmonary artery and in the proximal aorta, and the shunt volume is the difference between them (Figure 8.10)[17, 18].

8.6 Atrial Septal Defect

Atrial septal defect (ASD) consists in a defect in the interatrial septum that permits communication between both atria. Four types of ASD can be distinguished: 1) *Ostium secundum*, the most frequent, the defect being placed in the middle of the interatrial septum, in the region of the fossa ovalis. 2) *Ostium primum*, where the defect is located in the most caudal part of the interatrial septum and it is associated with anomalies of the atrioventricular valves, usually a cleft in the left atrioventricular valve, causing valve regurgitation. 3) *Sinus venosus*, although included among the ASDs, actually should be reagarded as an anomalous venous connection. The defect is located near the drainage of the venae cavae, most commonly it's placed in the cephalad part of the atrial septum, opposite the entry of the superior vena cava (superior vena cava defect), but sometimes it's being found posteriorly o posteroinferiorly to the fosa ovalis, near the entry of the inferior vena cava (inferior vena cava defect); in the superior vena cava type, an anomalous connection of right pulmonary veins, with a right

FIGURE 8.7

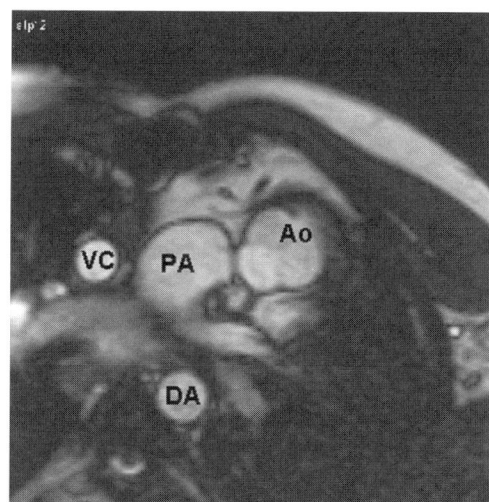 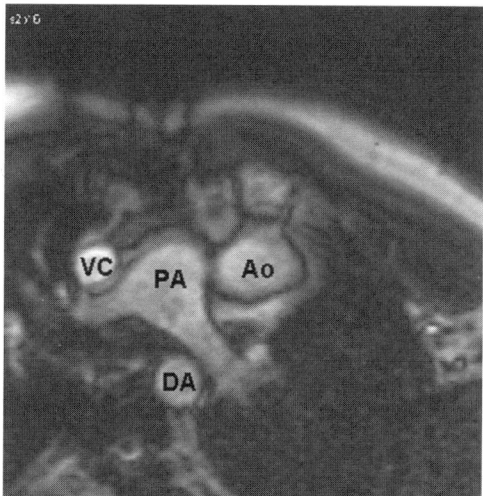

FIGURE 8.8

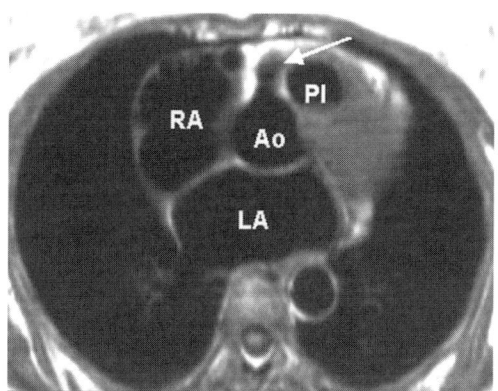 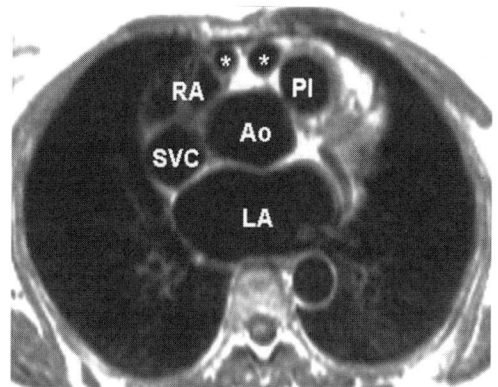

F. 8.7. Parallel axial planes on GRE showing the aortic root (Ao) situated anteriorly and to the left of the pulmonary artery (PA), which may be easily identificated by its early bifurcation (right panel). This relationship of the great arteries is known as L-transposition. VC: superior vena cava; DA: descending aorta.

F. 8.8. Patient with a right coronary fistula draining into the coronary sinus. Left panel: Axial T1w SE section showing a dilated proximal segment of the right coronary artery, with an anomalous origin and course, directed towards the anterior wall chest (arrow). Right panel: axial plane at a more cranial level than the previous one showing crossectional views of the tortuous course of the coronary fistula (asterisks) on the anterior aspect of the heart. Ao: aortic root; LA: left atrium; PI: pulmonary infundibulum; RA: right atrium; SVC: superior vena cava.

FIGURE 8.9

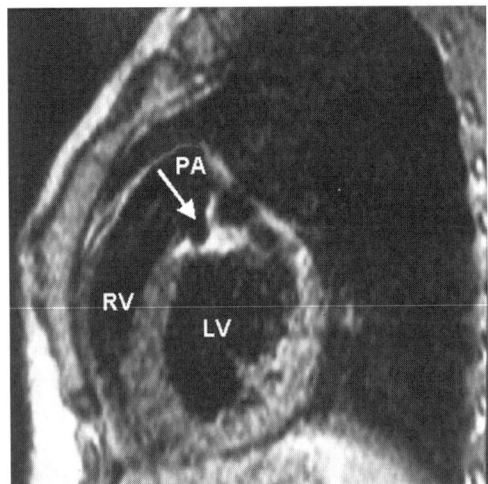

F. 8.9.   Sagittal T1w SE plane showing the origin of the left coronary artery (arrow) from the posterior wall of the main pulmonary artery (PA) in a case of anomalous origin of left coronary artery. LV: left ventricle; RV: right ventricle.

superior pulmonary vein emptying directly into the right atrium or into the superior vena cava, is frequently associated. 4) Coronary sinus type ASD: it is an infrequent anomaly characterized by a defect in the coronary sinus roof, which permits communication between the left atrium and the right atrium through the coronary sinus.

The volume of the interatrial shunt, usually left-to-right, with the consequent right ventricle volume overload and increased pulmonary flow, depends on the size of the defect, but specially on the end-diastolic ventricular pressure of both ventricles or, in other words, on the different compliance of both ventricular chambers.

CMR permits an easy evaluation of the size of the right cardiac chambers as well as the pulmonary arterial trunk and its main branches, giving indirect information about the volume of the shunt. Regarding morphological evaluation of the atrial septal defect, CMR is specially useful in the diagnosis of *sinus venosus* type, where transthoracic echocardiography may have diagnostic problems, particularly in adult patients. In these cases, CMR usually depicts the defect and also a frequently associated partial anomalous pulmonary venous connection to the superior vena cava, in the superior vena cava type (Figure 8.11), and to the inferior vena cava, in the inferior vena cava type. In

ostium secundum ASD, CMR, specially with old systems, may lead to false positive results due to the thinning of the fossa ovalis membrane, that may produce an apparent defect on the image of the interatrial septum; therefore, in these cases, special care should be taken and the atrial septum should be examined in various planes using, basically, axial slices (Figure 8.12)[19]. The visualization of flow through the defect, by cine MR, will help to confirm the diagnosis. Velocity-encoded cine CMR may be used to quantify stroke flow in the aorta and main pulmonary artery, and to estimate the shunt volume, by calculating the relation of flows (Qp:Qs) (Figure 8.10)[20, 21].

8.7   Ventricular Septal Defect

Ventricular septal defect (VSD) consists in an orifice in the interventricular septum. It may be small or large, restrictive or nonrestrictive to blood flow, single or multiple, and may be placed in several regions. The VSD is classified as: a) muscular, when the edges of the defect are totally composed of muscular tissue; b) perimembranous, when they are located around the membranous septum and the central fibrous body constitutes one of its edges; c) subarterial, when it is situated below the pulmonary and aortic valves and there is aortopulmonary continuity. Muscular defects and perimembranous ones can be subclassified according to their location at the level of the inlet septum (near atrioventricular valves), the trabecular septum, and/or the outlet septum. The volume of the shunt will be conditioned by the size of the VSD and the relationship between the pulmonary and the systemic vascular resistances. The progressive increase of the former will reduce the volume of the shunt even leading to its inversion. It should be noted that, in some cases, the valvular structures surrounding the defect may progressively limit its size. For example, in subtricuspidal defects, the growth of new fibrous tissue, coming from the tricuspid valve or from the membranous septum, may seal the defect. Likewise, in subaortic or subarterial perimembranous defects, the prolapse of the valve may progressively reduce the volume of the shunt ultimately closing the defect, but developing

FIGURE 8.10

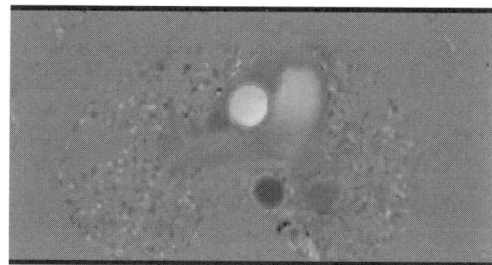 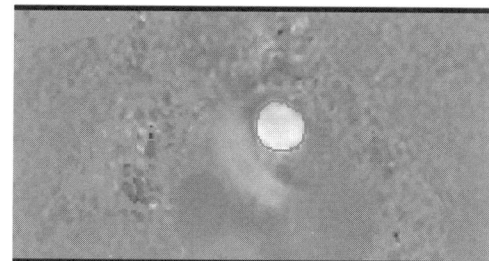

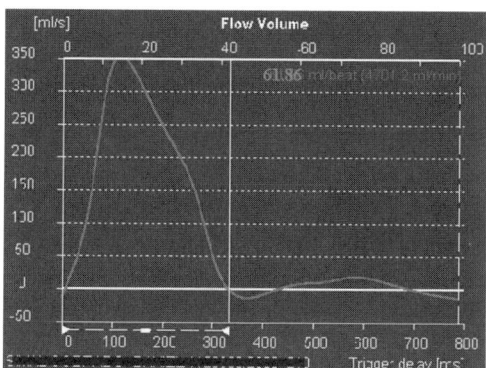 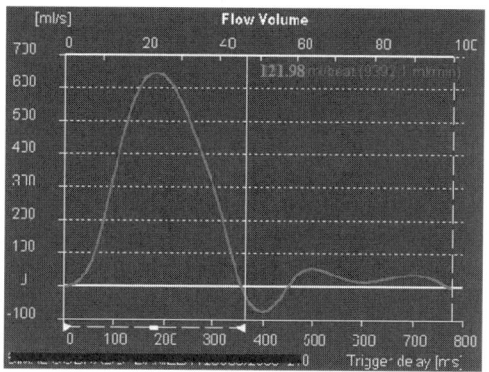

FIGURE 8.11

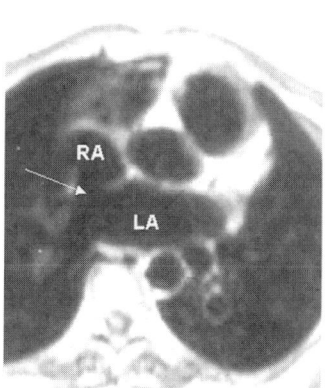 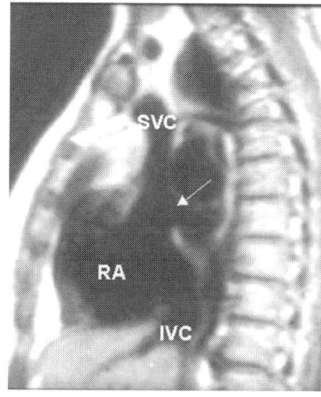 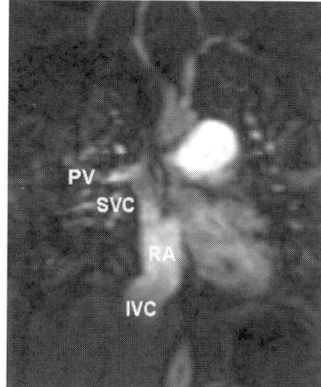

F. 8.10. Studies of flow velocity mapping at the ascending aorta (top left) and the pulmonary artery (top right) in a case of left-to-right shunt: volume curves show an aortic systolic flow of 61.86 ml (bottom left) and a pulmonic one of 121.98 ml, this indicating a Qp/Qs ratio = 2.

F. 8.11. Patient with a *sinus venosus* atrial septal defect, at level of the entry of the superior vena cava (SVC), visualized on both axial (left panel) and sagittal (middle panel) T1w SE planes (arrows). A coronal plane from an MRA contrast study on a different patient (right panel) with an atrial septal defect *sinus venosus* type shows a right pulmonary vein (PV) draining directly into the SVC. IVC: inferior vena cava; LA: left atrium; RA: right atrium.

FIGURE 8.12

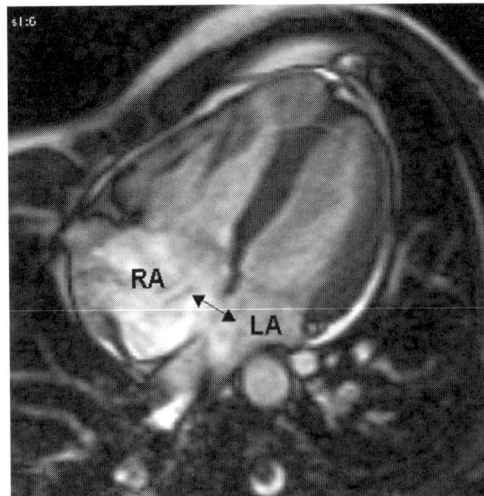 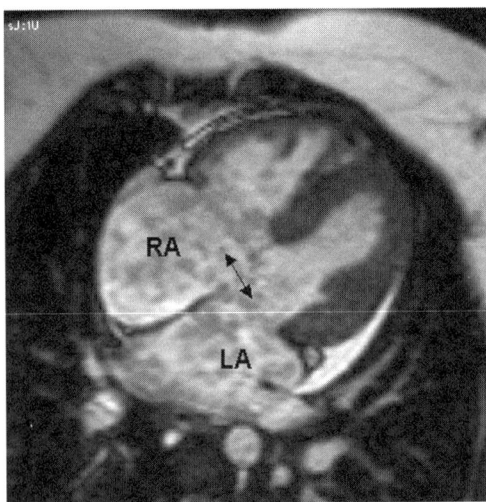

FIGURE 8.13

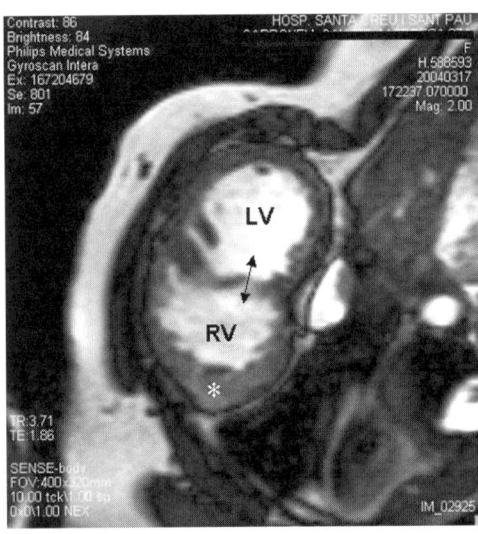 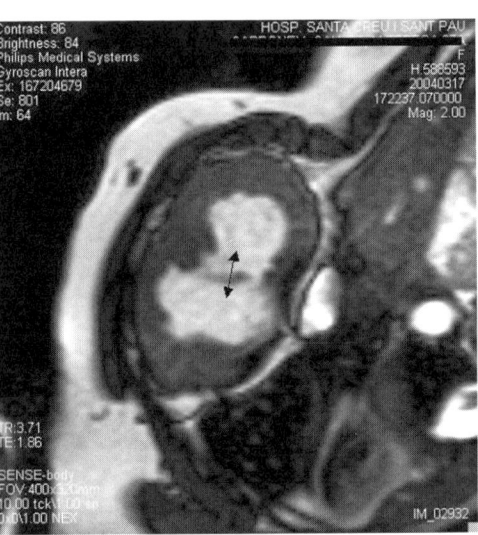

F. 8.12.   Horizontal longitudinal planes from cine sequences showing atrial septal defects (arrows) of the *ostium secundum* (left panel) and *ostium primum* (right panel) type. LA: left atrium; RA: right atrium.

F. 8.13.   Short axis diastolic (left panel) and systolic (right panel) images from a cine sequence in a patient with a large VSD (arrows). Note the marked hypertrophy of the right ventricular wall (asterisk) secondary to severe chronic pulmonary hypertension (Eisenmenger's syndrome). LV: left ventricle; RV: right ventricle.

aortic or pulmonary insufficiency, which in some cases can become severe and require a valvular prosthesis.

By using planes aligned orthogonally with the interventricular septum, SE or cine techniques may be used to visualize VSDs of moderate and large size[22] (Figure 8.13), but because of its resolution it is not useful in the study of small VSDs[23], specially the muscular ones. Defects in the trabecular portion can be visualized from any view: axial, coronal or sagittal. It is important to complete the morphological study of the VSD with cine CMR using GRE technique, because it will show the blood flow passing through the defect. When the defects are small, they may be diagnosed by visualization during systole of a signal loss in the right side of the interventricular septum, produced by the high velocity of the transorificial flow. Certainly, moving blood gives a high signal in cine MR, but in areas of turbulence the signal is lost. The outflow tract of the right ventricle should be analysed systematically to diagnose a possible infundibular or valvular pulmonary stenosis associated to the ventricular septal defect.

8.8 Atrioventricular Defects

They occur as a consequence of an anomalous development of the endocardial cushions, which causes a defect in the atrioventricular septum as well as anomalies in the atrioventricular valves. There are partial forms, as it is the *ostium primum* ASD, characterized by the absence of the inferior or caudal portion of the atrial septum and a ''cleft'' at level of the left atrioventricular valve, causing regurgitation, and complete forms, made up of an atrial septal defect type *ostium primum* which extends down into the ventricular septum, and a single atrioventricular valve (complete atrioventricular canal). Between these two types, there are intermediate forms. All types of atrioventricular defects share the absence of the atrioventricular septum, lying both atrio-ventricular valves at the same level (Figure 8.12, right panel).

Using SE CMR to study the four chamber with axial planes (usually with a slight oblique angulation), the absence of the normal insertion of the atrioventricular valves at two different levels into the interventricular septum, as well as the septal defects, can be observed. Nevertheless, in the majority of patients, this information can also be obtained by echocardiography. Therefore, CMR should be reserved for specific cases where diagnostic doubts persist. For example, to evaluate a possible small ventricular septal defect associated to an atrial septal defect with a single atrioventricular valve. In the last case, coronal slices with a slight obliquity can help in the diagnosis. Likewise, as CMR provides a wide view of thoracic structures, it is also a good method to evaluate the size of heart chambers, allowing the detection of a possible disproportion of sizes among them, mainly between both ventricles, with dominance of either the morphologically left or right ventricle[24, 25]. This is especially important when a surgical correction is being evaluated, as the risk is higher and the results usually worst in cases with ventricular hypoplasia. Cine CMR may be useful to evaluate valve function. Sometimes it may give more information than echocardiography about blood jet direction and its consequences. For example, in cases of *ostium primum* atrial septal defect, the left atrioventricular valve regurgitation may be directed toward the right atrium throught the atrial septal defect. There is a mandatory shunt from the left ventricle to the right atrium, which may be responsible of early clinical symptomatology.

8.9 Patent Ductus Arteriosus

The ductus arteriosus, the most common type of extracardiac shunt, represents persistent patency of the vessel that normally connects in the fetus the pulmonary artery and the aorta, 5–10 mm below the origin of the left subclavian artery. It usually obliterates after birth, firstly by contraction of the medial smooth muscle (functional closure) and later by connective tissue formation and fibrosis. By 2–3 weeks the closure is completed. If the vessel remains open, a shunt results, normally left-to-right, from the aorta to the pulmonary artery. This anomaly is called patent o persistent ductus arteriosus (PDA). If the pulmonary flow is significantly increased, a dilatation of the left chambers and the ascending aorta will result. Children with a large PDA may show a progressive elevation in pulmonary vascular resistence, as a consequence of the development of a pulmonary vasculopathy, eventually resulting in reversal of the shunt and differential cyanosis (cyanosis in the inferior limbs with a more rose-colored coloration in the superior limbs, corresponding to Eisenmenger's syndrome).

In small children, PDA can be usually diagnosed by 2D-Doppler echocardiography, but this may be difficult in adult patients. It is in these cases where CMR can be useful,[26, 27] using the SE technique and in coronal or sagittal planes with a slight obliquity (Figure 8.14), or, even better, using cine CMR. If the ductus is small, short or tortuous, CMR can give rise to a false negative.

FIGURE 8.14

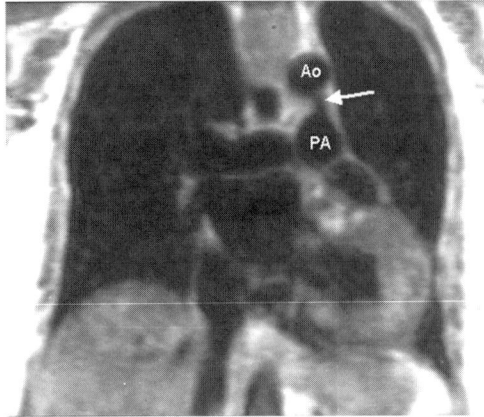

F. 8.14. Coronal plane showing the presence of a patent ductus arteriosus (arrow) connecting the aorta (Ao) and the main pulmonary artery (PA).

8.10   Obstructive Lesions

Valvular stenosis is discussed in another section of this book (Chapter 5), the basic concepts explained there being also applicable to congenital valvular stenosis.[28] This section will be specifically dedicated to the study of: 1) right ventricular outflow obstruction, 2) valvular and supravalvular pulmonary stenosis, 3) fixed subvalvular and supravalvular aortic stenosis, and 4) coarctation of the aorta.

a. Right ventricular outflow tract obstruction

CMR is very useful for the morphological analysis of the myocardium. It may easily visualize a hypertrophied right ventricle helping also in identifying the distribution of hypertrophy: i.e.: diffuse, shaped by ventricular bands, or located at the infundibular level, with the consequent obstruction to ventricular ejection[29] (see the section on Tetralogy of Fallot). The measurement of blood velocity by phase mapping techniques permits to calculate the gradient, as it may be accomplished by conventional Doppler techniques. Infundibular obstruction will be better observed in coronal planes or in those oblique planes that can be aligned longitudinally with the right ventricular outflow tract.

b. Valvular and supravalvular pulmonary stenosis

Pulmonary valve morphology is not easily assessed using CMR. Only thickened and dysplasic valves with restricted opening, can be visualized with MR, especially using the SE technique. It is easier to detect an hypertrophied right ventricle, with a possible associated infundibular obstruction, as well as a post-stenotic dilated pulmonary arterial trunk.[30] By means of the typical image of signal void, the GRE technique permits to visualize a turbulent flow at valvular or subvalvular level. If velocity phase mapping is available, the valvular or subvalvular pulmonary gradient can be calculated.

Supravalvular stenosis, generally ring-shaped, can be located above the valve, at the level of the pulmonary arterial trunk, which shows an hour-glass shaped morphology, or at the level of the distal pulmonary branches, being usually multiple. In the latter cases, their visualization by CMR can be difficult, and for the diagnosis could be necessary to look for the narrowing of the flow signal or the signal loss using the GRE technique.

c. Subvalvular and supravalvular aortic stenosis

Dynamic obstruction of the left ventricular outflow is discussed in the Chapter dealing with cardiomyopathies; therefore, only subvalvular fixed stenosis will be studied here. These can consist of a fibrous or fibromuscular ring, or may be more diffuse, presenting as a true tunnel throughout the outflow tract. These anomalies are usually diagnosed by echocardiography. Nevertheless, in cases with a difficult echocardiographic window, CMR SE technique using oblique slices similar to the left anterior oblique projection in angiography can be useful to study subaortic morphology. At the same time it provides information about the degree of secondary hypertrophy of the left ventricle. The GRE technique will confirm the level of obstruction, and the flow analysis by velocity mapping will permit calculation of the gradient.

Supravalvular stenosis, normally consisting of a fibrous ring near the aortic valve, is much less frequent. In contrast with aortic subvalvular stenosis, CMR plays an important role in its study. It can provide morphological information by means of the SE technique and functional information by means of velocity mapping.

d. Coarctation of the aorta

Coarctation of the aorta consists on a constriction of the aortic lumen, usually discrete, sometimes of significant length, generally located at the beginning of the descending aorta, after the origin of the left subclavian artery, but in rare cases placed at level of aortic arch or even at the abdominal aorta. Mainly in old children, adolescents and adults, large collateral vessels develop from the subclavian artery through the internal mammary and intercostal arteries to the post-coarctation segment of the proximal descending aorta to give the classic sign of rib notching on the chest roentgenogram.

CMR is the non invasive preferred technique to demonstrate and evaluate a suspected coarctation of the aorta in older children, adolescents and adults[31], as is the case in other anomalies of the aortic arch (Figure 8.15). Certainly, echocardiography may fail in adequately displaying the lesion. CMR in SE or GRE (cine CMR) techniques, may locate the lesion, showing its morphology, length and severity (Figure 8.16), the size of the aortic isthmus and the aorta at the pre- and post-coarctation levels. CMR angiography techniques constitute, as in every aspect of aortic diseases, an important diagnostic tool in coarctation. In addition to the visualization of the defect in 3D mode, associated features as a possible aberrant subclavian artery, or collateral vessels, as dilated intercostals arteries running along the underside of the posterior upper ribs, or dilated internal mammary arteries along the anterior chest wall, can also be displayed (Figure 8.17).

Using phase-contrast CMR, is possible to measure the flow through the collateral arteries by comparing flow volume just distal to the stenosis with flow volume through the descending aorta at the diaphragmatic level (Figure 8.18). In moderate to severe aortic coarctation, an increase in flow volume of approximately 80% can be observed, whereas in normals usually a 7% decrease is detected[32].

In summary, together with the external gradient (difference in systolic arterial pressure between the superior and inferior limbs), easily mesurable at the physical exam, CMR provides all the necessary information in aortic coarctation prior to surgery.[33]

The best views are usually the axial and oblique ones, specifically the oblique left anterior. Attempts must be always made to obtain a slice aligned longitudinally with the coarctated area. Incorrect alignments can give rise to false positives or to exaggerate the severity of the obstruction.

As a consequence of its high anatomical resolution, CMR is also the best technique to evaluate the surgical results, independently of the type of surgery (resection and end-to-end anastomosis, patch, tubular graft, etc.) (Figure 8.19), or the results of balloon catheter angioplasty with o without stent implantation. Residual stenosis, recoarctation, o possible complications related with the therapeutic procedure used (aortic aneurysm, aortic dissection, periaortic hematoma), can be easily detected.

8.11 Complex Congenital Heart Diseases

Complex congenital heart lesions refer to anomalies characterized by the association of various defects. Some associations may be even necessary, in a particular case, for the development to term of the fetus. In order to consider eventual surgery and/or to make a prognosis, it is necessary to identify all of the lesions. CMR usually provides important morphological and functional information, but in order to complete the study, it is used in combination with echocardiography and, frequently, with cardiac catherization. Some of these anomalies will be described in the next paragraphs.

a. Tetralogy of Fallot

Fallot's Tetralogy is the most frequent cyanotic congenital heart disease, especially in patients over two years of age. It basically consists of: a) extensive subaortic ventricular septal defect (malalignement VSD); b) dextroposition of the aorta origin; c) infundibular pulmonary stenosis; d) right ventricular hypertrophy (Figure 8.20). Other frequently associated anomalies are: valvular pulmonary stenosis,

FIGURE 8.15

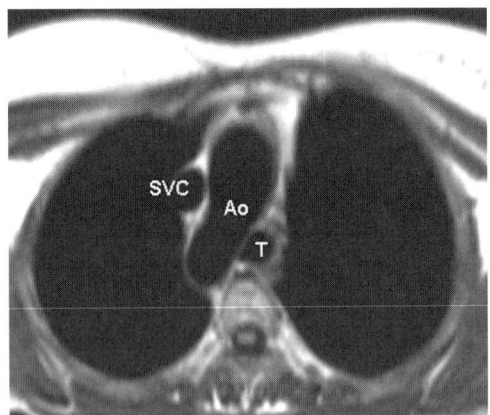 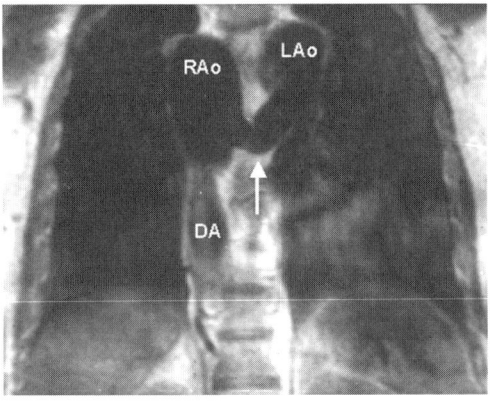

FIGURE 8.16

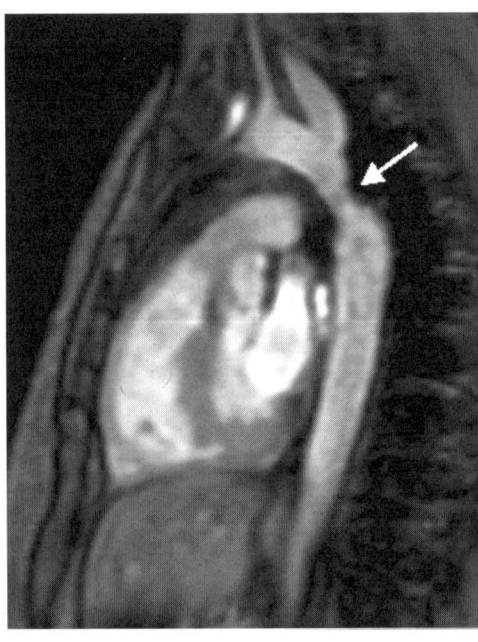 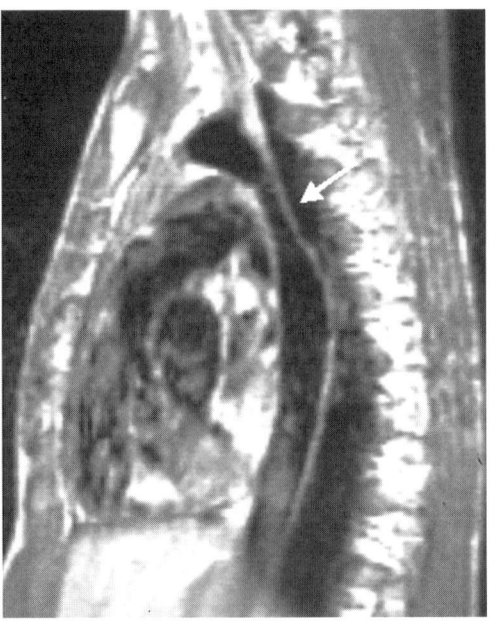

F. 8.15. Left panel: Axial T1w SE plane in a case of right aortic arch (Ao) situated between the trachea (T) and the superior vena cava (SVC). Right panel: Coronal T1w SE plane showing a double aortic arch, right (RAo) and left (LAo), and their union (arrow) to form a single descending aorta (DA).

F. 8.16. Left panel: Sagittal GRE image showing a classical form of aortic coarctation (arrow). Right panel: Sagittal T1w SE in a case of tubular form of coarctation (arrow).

F. 8.17. Maximum intensity projection (MIP) image from a CMR contrast angiography of the aorta showing coarctation (black arrow) and an extense system of collateral vessels involving the mammary arteries (white short arrow) and the intercostals arteries (white long arrow).

F. 8.18. Study of collateral flow volume in aortic coarctation by means of phase velocity sequences. Left panel: levels of interrogation at the descending aorta: proximal, immediately below the coarctation (upper line), and distal, at the diaphragmatic aorta (lower line). Middle panel: corresponding crossections of the aorta. Right panel: flow curves from the proximal (solid) and distal (broken) descending aorta; the increased flow volume at the distal level is due to the collateral flow.

F. 8.19. MIP images from CMR angiography contrast studies in patients with surgically corrected coarctation. On the left panel, only a mild indentation in the aortic wall (arrow) is visualized after a patch repair; on the right, a tubular graft is seen (arrow) bypassing the coarctation.

FIGURE 8.17

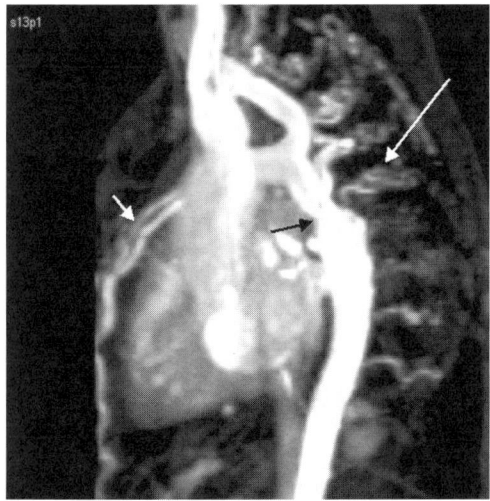

FIGURE 8.18

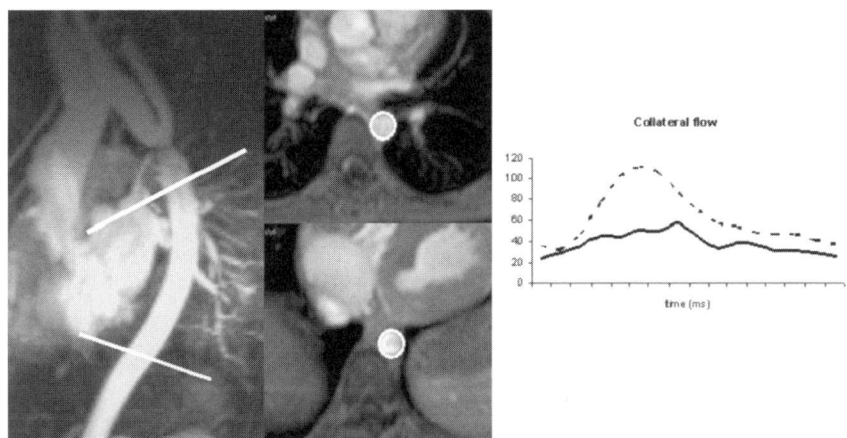

FIGURE 8.19

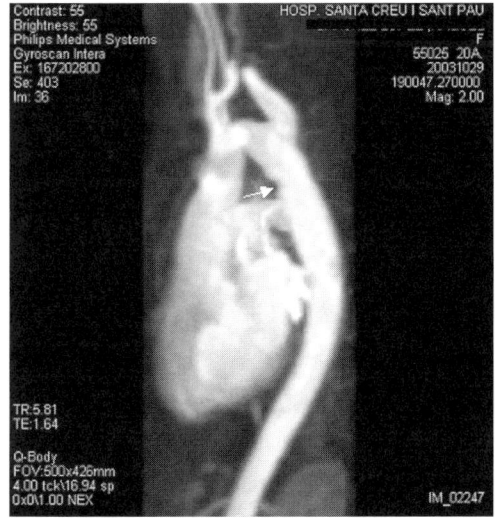
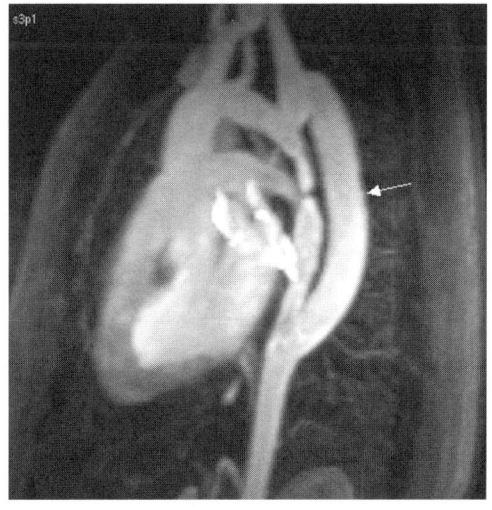

FIGURE 8.20

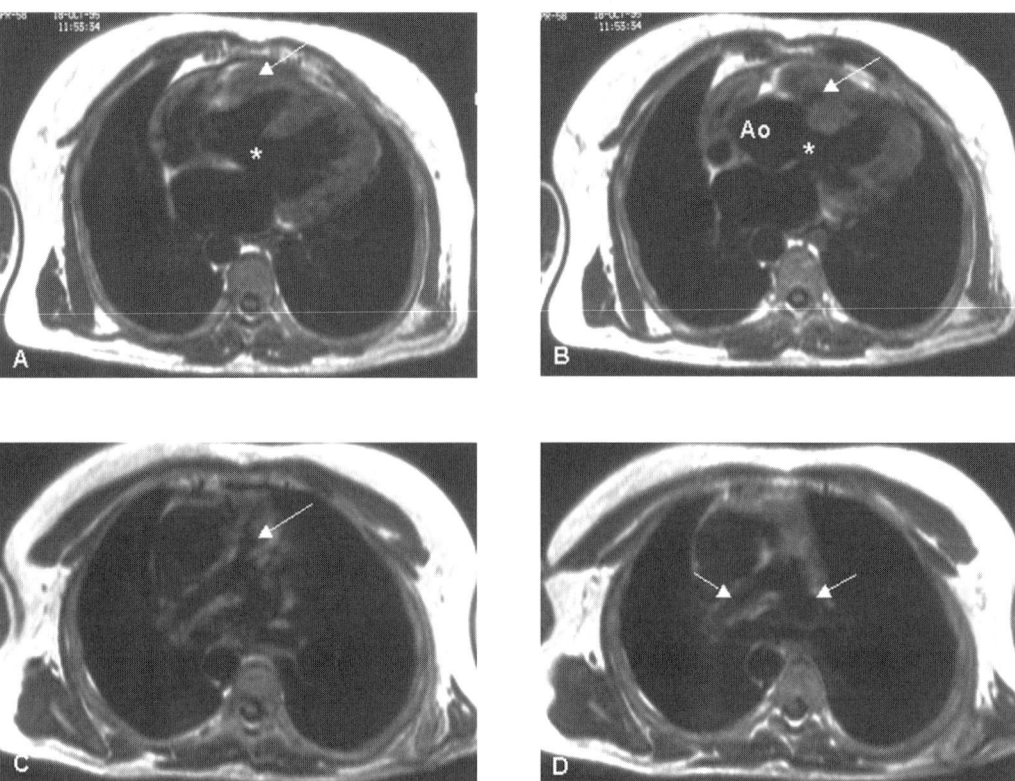

F. 8.20. Features of tetralogy of Fallot in CMR. Axial T1w SE sequences from the same patient, in ascending caudo-cranial order, from A to D. A: right ventricular hypertrophy (arrow), and interventricular septal defect (asterisk). B: aorta (Ao) straddling over the ventricular defect (asterisk), and severe pulmonary infundibular stenosis (arrow). C: moderate hypoplasia of the main pulmonary artery (arrow). D: normal size of both pulmonary artery branches.

stenosis of the pulmonary branches, right aortic arch, atrial septal defect, anomalies in the origin and course of the coronary arteries, etc. The treatment of this anomaly requires surgery, either palliative or corrective. The shunting operations (palliative) increase pulmonary flow, but they should be regarded as preliminary to more complete correction. The more usual surgical shunt is the Blalock-Taussig fistula, which connects the subclavian artery with the pulmonary artery . Anatomical correction consists on closing the ventricular septal defect by a patch, and on relieving the infundibular stenosis by excision of the obstructing muscle bundles. In cases of associated pulmonary valve stenosis, it will be necessary to practice a pulmonary valvotomy. If the obstruction remains incompletely relieved, an outflow patch may be incorporated to the ventriculotomy closure enlarging the ventricular outflow. When the pulmonary annulus and the main pulmonary artery are

small, the patch may be extended from the infundibulum to the pulmonary artery trunk (transannular patch), but that may cause an important pulmonic regurgitation, that may be well tolerated in the short and medium term, but may result in right ventricular failure, arrhythmias, and sudden death some years after surgery.

CMR can be useful for the study of the Tetralogy of Fallot, before and after surgery, providing additional information to that rendered by echocardiography.[34] Except in those cases with poor echocardiographic windows, the basic lesions can be easily visualized by using either one of both techniques. However, CMR has proved to be superior to echocardiography in evaluating many other important aspects, as the size of the pulmonary arterial trunk and its branches (Figure 8.21), its growth following palliative surgery (an important data when posterior corrective surgery is under consideration), the presence of supravalvular pulmonary stenosis, or right ventricular outflow tract aneurysm, and, specially, in evaluating the presence and severity of pulmonary valve regurgitation, and the right and left ventricular function. Certainly, an important issue after correction of tetralogy of Fallot is the quantification of pulmonary regurgitation (Figure 8.22) and its influence on the function of the right ventricle. Left ventricular dysfunction has been correlated with right ventricular dysfunction, through an unfavourable interaction between the ventricles (Figure 8.23), both having been associated with poor outcome[35]. CMR has emerged as the gold standard for the study of these parameters (see Chapter 2).

The origin and course of the coronary arteries is an important point where echocardiography usually fails, and although CMR may be useful, not unfrequently a cardiac catheterization is required before corrective surgery.

To study Fallot's Tetralogy by CMR, sections in different planes should be made: axial, sagittal, coronal, and sometimes obliques, as are those transversal slices with ascending obliquity in an antero-posterior projection (similar to the sitting-up plane in angiography), useful to study the pulmonary arterial trunk and its main branches. By GRE CMR it is easy to detect hypoplasia of these branches, since it permits to distinguish them from the adjacent bronchi. As a general rule, the left pulmonary artery runs above the main left bronchus, which is posterior to the left pulmonary veins. On the right side, the main right bronchus is posterior to the right pulmonary artery, while the pulmonary veins are placed anteriorly and inferiorly. It should be noted that, when a pulmonary artery is absent, a GRE study also facilitates the diagnosis (Figure 8.24).

b. Truncus arteriosus

It consists on the presence of a single vessel straddling a ventricular septal defect and from which, the aorta, the coronary arteries, and the pulmonary artery arise. This vessel collects the blood from both ventricles. There are different types of truncus arteriosus, depending on the way in which the pulmonary arteries originate. In Type I, a short main pulmonary artery arises from the truncus, and gives rise to left and right pulmonary artery. In Types II and III, there is not a main pulmonary artery, the right and left branches arising directly from the common trunk. In Type IV, there is absence of pulmonary arteries, the lungs being supplied by large aortopulmonary collateral arteries. Nowadays, Type IV is considered to be a variant of pulmonary atresia with ventricular septal defect. The identification of all these vessels is very important, both for the classification of the anomaly and for the evaluation of the possible surgical alternatives.

Pulmonary atresia with ventricular septal defect is a congenital heart anomaly characterized by absence of connection between the right ventricle and the pulmonary arteries, associated with a ventricular septal defect and a biventricular heart. The lungs will be supplied from a patent ductus and/or from major aortopulmonary collaterals (MAPCA) coming off from the descending aorta below the isthmus and, sometimes, from the subclavian arteries. Pulmonary artery development varies from complete absence, or hypoplasia of all central pulmonary arteries, to completely developed pulmonary arteries beyond an atretic but imperforate pulmonary valve. Sometimes, the trunk or a branch of the pulmonary artery may be absent, or the trunk may be not connected to a pulmonary branch, etc. Actually, the pulmonary vascularization can be extraordinarily anomalous. In order to evaluate the feasibility of surgical repair of this anomaly, one of the most important issues is to demonstrate the central confluence and the adequate size of the right and left pulmonary artery, even when the main pulmonary artery is atretic. The visualization of aorto-pulmonary collaterals is difficult, even using angiography, but crucial for surgery in order to close them during the procedure.

The use of CMR can provide important anatomic information about any type of truncus[36] (Figure 8.25 and 8.26) as well as about pulmonary atresia with ventricular septal defect. It is necessary to evaluate different planes for the complete study of the pulmonary arteries, and especially of the aorto-pulmonary collaterals (Figure 8.27 and 8.28)[37].

c. Complete transposition of the great arteries

This anomaly is characterized by the association of atrioventricular concordance with ventriculoarterial discordance. The anatomical

FIGURE 8.21

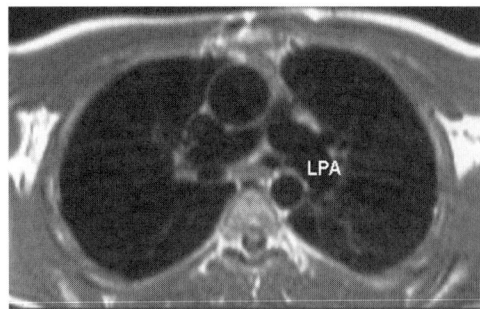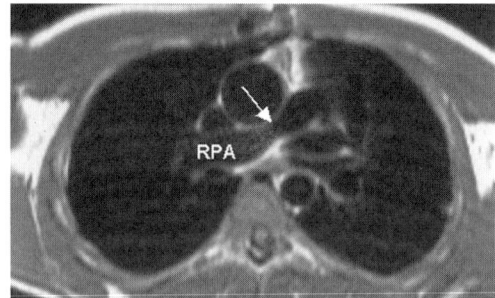

FIGURE 8.22

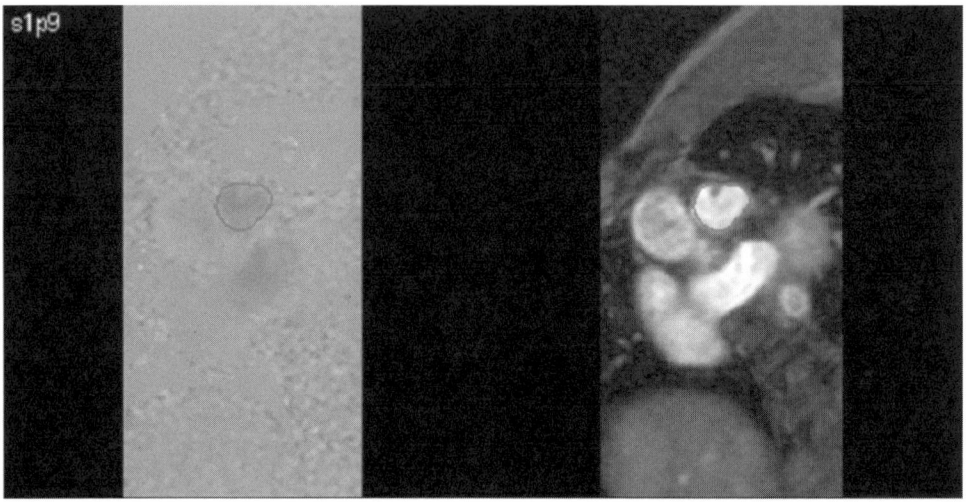

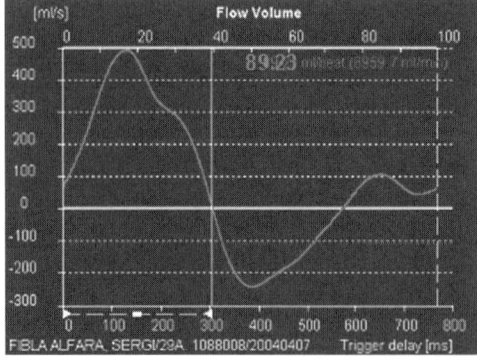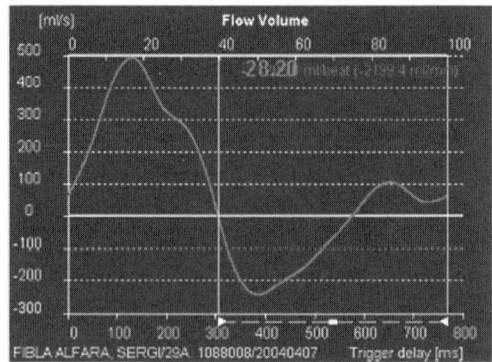

F. 8.21. Axial T1w SE images from a patient with a surgically corrected tetralogy of Fallot showing, on the left panel, a left pulmonary artery (LPA) of normal size and regular shape, while, on the right panel, a moderate reduction in the diameter (arrow) of the right pulmonary artery (RPA) is seen.

F. 8.22. Top: Phase velocity (left) and amplitude (right) images from the main pulmonary artery (manually traced) in a case of pulmonary insufficiency after repair of Fallot's tetralogy. Bottom: flow-velocity curve where the antegrade systolic (left) and the retrograde diastolic (right) flows have been calculated, a regurgitant fraction of 32% being estimated.

F. 8.23. Short axis cine sequences in two patients with surgically corrected Fallot's tetralogy. Top: diastolic (left) and systolic (right) images showing a patch at the right ventricular infundibulum (arrows), with preserved contractile function of the remaining right ventricle (RV), and also of the left ventricle (LV). Bottom: diastolic (left) and systolic (right) frames from another patient, in this case showing depressed systolic function of both the right (RV) and left (LV) ventricles.

F. 8.24. Axial GRE image in a patient with Fallot's tetralogy and absence of the right pulmonary artery (asterisk); in addition, there is also a right aortic arch: note the descending aorta (DA) situated to the right of the vertebral column. AA: ascending aorta; LPA: left pulmonary artery; MPA: main pulmonary artery; SVC: superior vena cava.

FIGURE 8.23

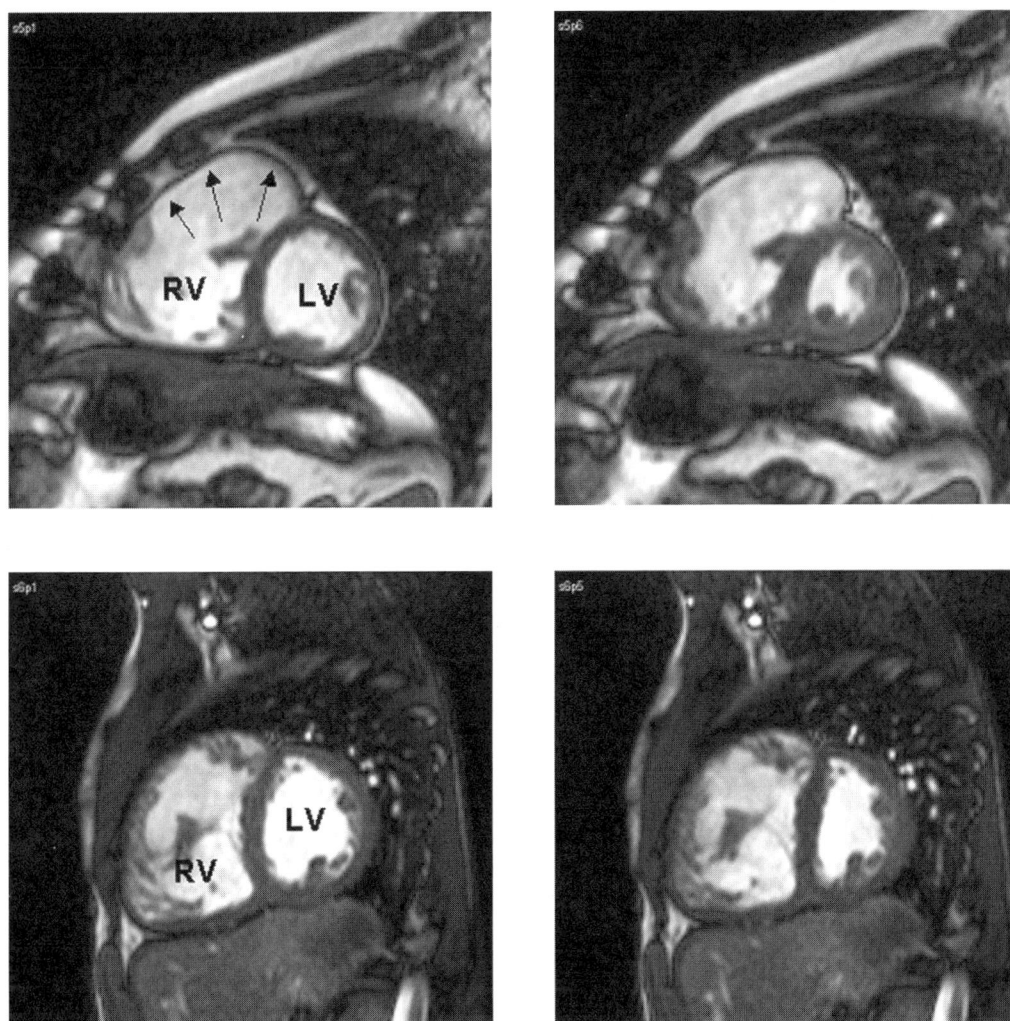

FIGURE 8.24

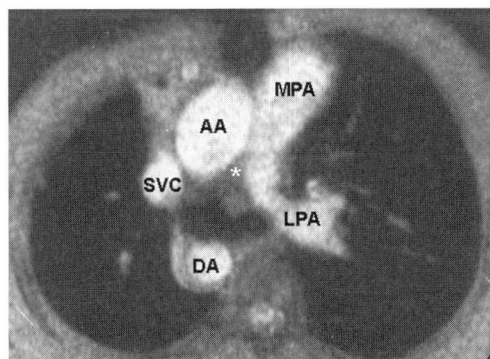

arrangement results in two separate and parallel circulations. Some communication between both circulations is necessary for survival. The minimum communications which permit subsistence of the newborn are the foramen ovale and the ductus arteriosus, but they tend to close in the first few days of life, being necessary to perform some paliative technique, as a transcatheter balloon atrial septostomy, and/or a corrective operation.

In the most common type of complete transposition of the great arteries, the aortic valve (and the initial portion of the ascending aorta) is usually placed in front of and to the right of the pulmonary valve, a position which is known as D-transposition. The aorta and the pulmonary artery do not cross, but they rather run parallel. The most frequent associated anomalies are ventricular septal defect (30% of the cases) and pulmonary stenosis.

Although the diagnosis is usually accomplished by echocardiography in the first week of life, CMR can be very useful to study children or adult patients, after an atrial (venous) or an arterial switch operation and in order to evaluate some residual lesions or sequelas o complications from the operation. Axial slices help in diagnosing the position of the arteries and in their identification. Coronal planes usually allow good visualization of the ventriculoarterial connection, while sagittal planes display the antero-posterior relationship of the great vessels. The latter ones are especially useful in order to demonstrate the origin of the aorta from the right ventricle (Figures 8.29 and 8.30). Associated anomalies, mainly ventricular septal defect or/and pulmonary stenosis may be demonstrated in axial and coronal planes. In patients undergoing physiological surgical correction (the systemic venous return is diverted into the left ventricle through the mitral valve, and then to the pulmonary artery, while the pulmonary venous return is diverted through the tricuspid valve to the right ventricle and the aorta), whether by the Mustard[38] or Senning[39] technique, CMR allows the study of a possible obstruction at level of the systemic or the pulmonary venous return, which is one of the most frequent complication in this type of surgical repair. The use in these patients of pulsed Doppler with CMR provides the greatest sensitivity and specificity for the detection of an obstruction in the drainage of the superior vena cava.[40]

Likewise, using the SE, and cine MR, it is possible to study the right ventricular function and to calculate the ejection fraction, which is an important data, as in these cases the right ventricle works as a systemic ventricle. In those patients who have been submitted to a Jatene type of anatomic correction[41] (arterial switch), CMR is useful to study the new ventriculoarterial connection (Figure 8.31 and 8.32), allowing to diagnose a possible supravalvular pulmonary stenosis and to detect possible valvular regurgitations, specially aortic regurgitation, as well as a decreased ventricular function, by using cine-CMR.

d. Tricuspid atresia

Tricuspid atresia is characterized by the absence of the right atrioventricular valve. It should be differentiated from cases with an imperforated tricuspid valve. In 65% of the cases, blood reaches the left atrium through a patent foramen ovale, and in the remaining cases through an atrial septal defect. In the most common type, it is associated with atrioventricular and ventriculoarterial concordance, and the flow that reaches the left ventricle is diverted to the aorta and to the the right ventricle through a ventricular septal defect (called bulboventricular foramen, as tricuspid atresia is considered a type of single ventricle with absence of the right atrioventricular connexion). The size of the right ventricle and the pulmonary artery depends primarily on the pulmonary flow, which is related to the size of the bulboventricular foramen as well as the presence of an associated infudibular or valvular pulmonary stenosis, that occurs in approximately 15% of the cases. There are other types of tricuspid atresia, such as the one associated with ventriculoarterial discordance or the one which presents discordant atrioventricular connection and double outlet of the morphologically right ventricle, generally associated with juxtaposition of the atrial appendages. The presence of pulmonary atresia with the aorta arising from the single ventricle as a single vessel is less frequent. In the more typical form, a left ventricle of normal size or enlarged and a small-sized chamber corresponding to the right ventricle can be seen in axial planes using SE MR. The chamber is usually located in an anterior and right position, separated from the

FIGURE 8.25

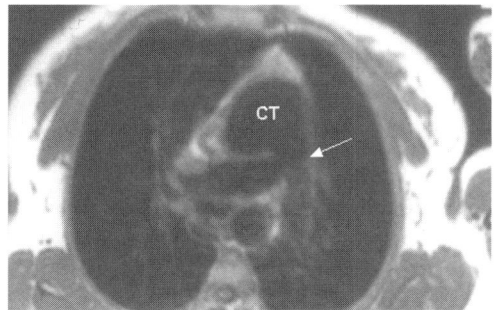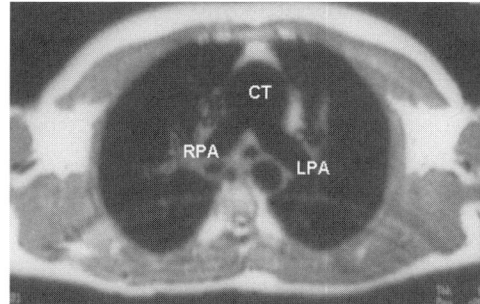

FIGURE 8.26

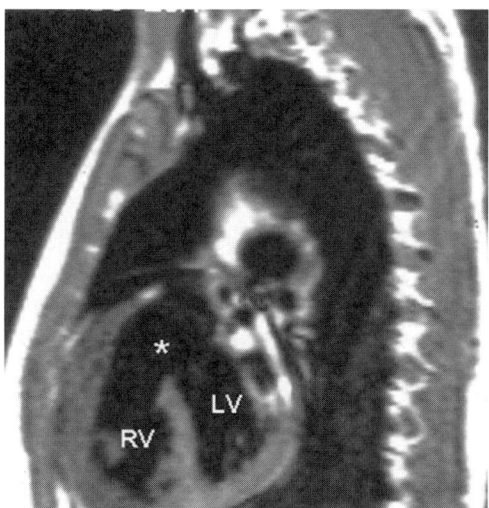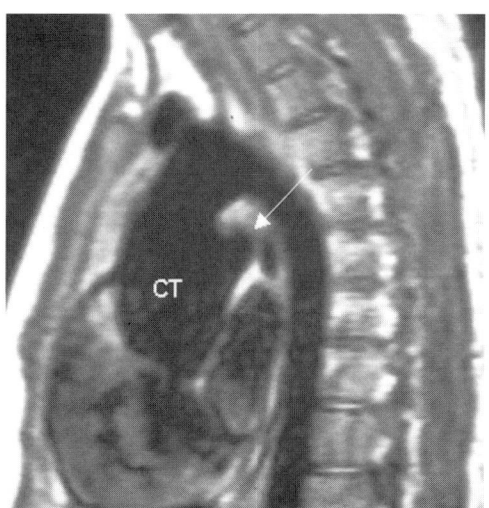

FIGURE 8.27

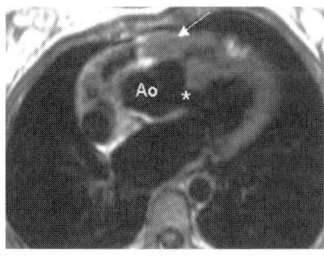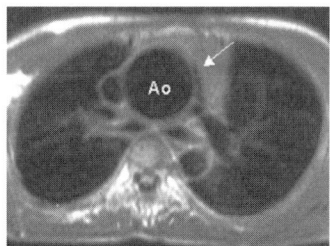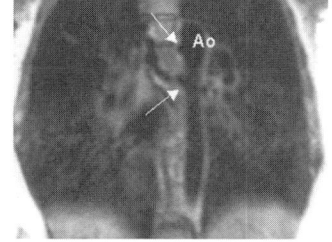

F. 8.25.　Axial T1w SE images from two patients with truncus arteriosus. Left: type I, with a short main pulmonary artery (arrow) arising from the common trunk (CT). Right: type II, where both the right (RPA) and left (LPA) pulmonary arteries arise independently from the CT..

F. 8.26.　Sagittal T1w SE images from a patient with truncus arteriosus. Left panel: a large defect (asterisk) is seen connecting both the right (RV) and left (LV) ventricles. Right panel: the main pulmonary artery is seen (arrow) arising from the common trunk (CT), proving the case to be a type I truncus arteriosus.

F. 8.27.　Features of pulmonary atresia at CMR. Left panel: axial T1w SE plane at the level of the ventricles showing that the pulmonary infundibulum is virtually absent (arrow), and a subaortic ventricular septal defect (asterisk). Middle panel: plane at the level of the great vessels, with an extremely hypoplastic main pulmonary trunk (arrow). Right panel: coronal plane showing major aorto-pulmonary collateral arteries (arrows). Ao: aorta.

FIGURE 8.28

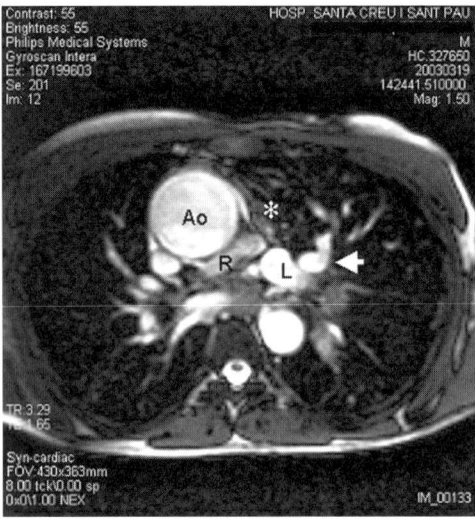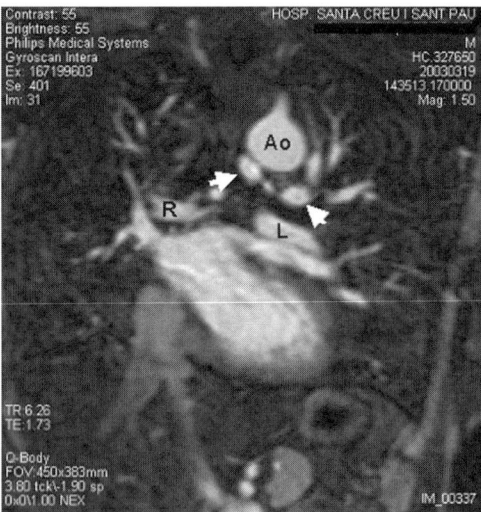

FIGURE 8.29

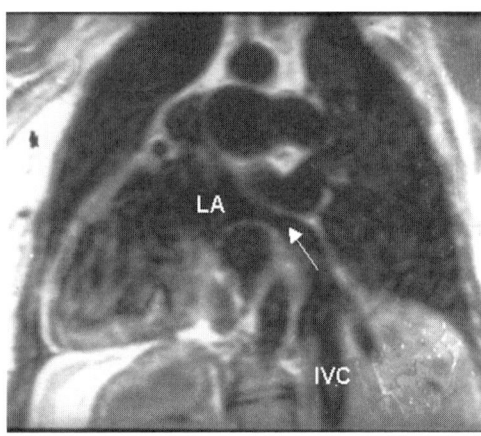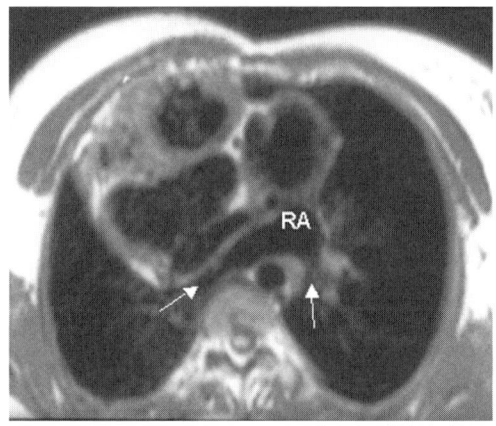

FIGURE 8.30

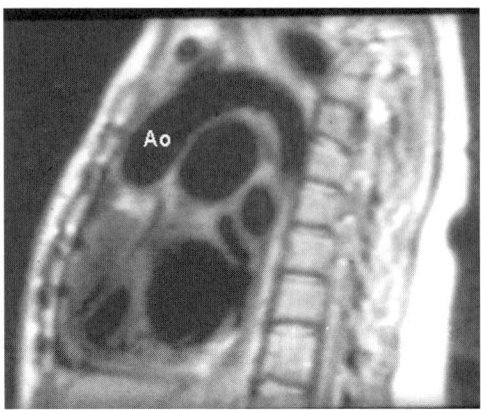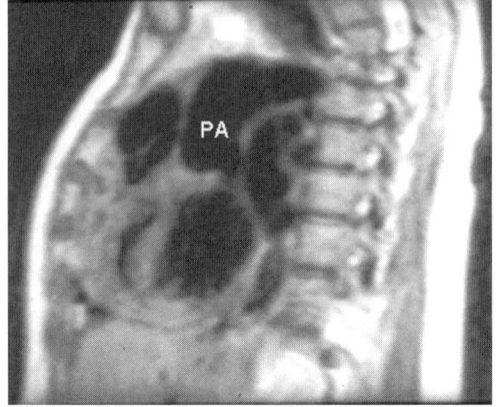

F. 8.28. Axial (left) and coronal (right) "bright-blood" GRE sequences from a patient with pulmonary atresia. Despite of the absence of pulmonary artery trunk (asterisk), non-confluent right (R) and left (L) pulmonary arterial branches are visualized, together with well-developped major aorto-pulmonary collateral arteries (arrows). Ao: aorta.

F. 8.29. Patient with transposition of the great arteries who had been submitted to an atrial shift operation (Mustard type). Left: coronal T1w SE plane showing a left-sided inferior vena cava (IVC) (*situs inversus*) which flow has been surgically re-directed (arrow) to the left atrium (LA). Right: axial T1w SE plane showing the surgically created drainage of the pulmonary veins (arrows) into the morphological right atrium (RA).

F. 8.30. Sagittal T1w SE planes from the same patient than in Figure 8.29. Left: the ascending aorta (Ao) is seen in an anterior position. Right: in this section, obtained somewhat rightward in relation to the previous one, the main pulmonary artery is seen in a posterior position.

FIGURE 8.31

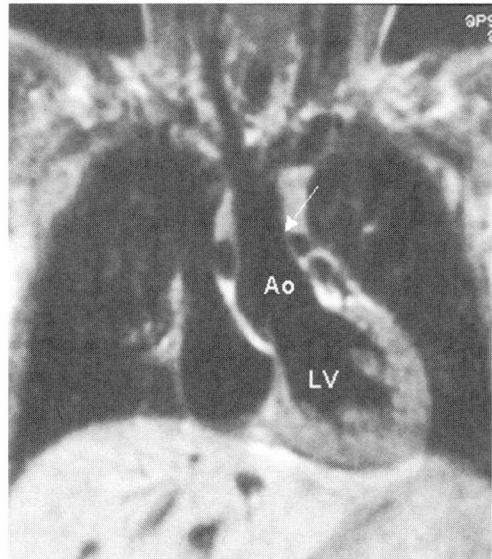 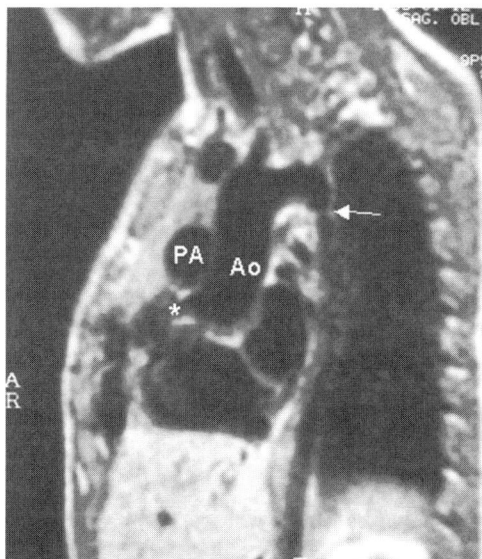

FIGURE 8.32

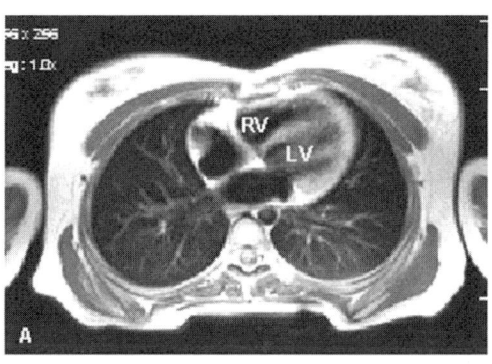 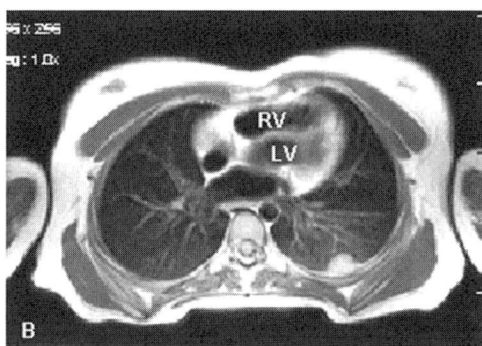

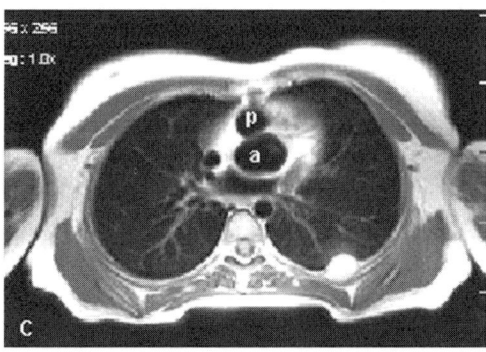 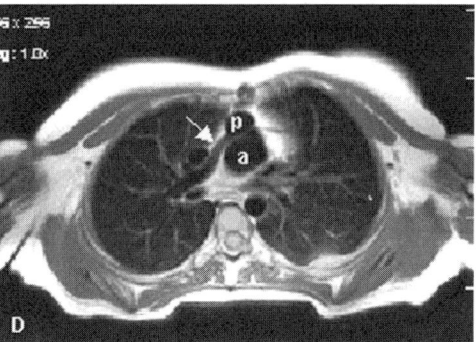

F. 8.31. Jatene operation (arterial switch) in a patient with complete D-transposition of the great arteries (atrioventricular concordance with ventriculoarterial discordance). Left: Coronal T1w SE plane showing the new emergence of the aorta (Ao) from the morphologically left ventricle (LV). Note the relatively abrupt reduction of the aorta at level of the anastomosis (arrow). Right: Oblique sagittal plane that shows the shape adopted by the aorta after being relocated in a position posterior to the pulmonary artery (PA). An aortic coarctation (arrow) can be observed at the beginning of the descending aorta. This lesion was not diagnosed prior to the surgical arterial switch, performed in the neonatal period. See the new origin of the right coronary artery (asterisk), which is dilated and without stenosis at this level.

F. 8.32. Axial "black-blood" SE images on ascending caudo-cranial order, from A to D, in a patient with transposition submitted to an arterial switch (Jatene's correction). The aorta (a) emerges from the left ventricle (LV), while the pulmonary artery (p) arises from the right ventricle (RV), a thin elongated right pulmonary artery being visualized (arrow in D).

right atrium, which appears to be potentially connected to the left ventricle, which supports, as we have previously mentioned, that some authors clasiffy this anomaly as a type of double atrio-ventricular inlet or single ventricle with atresia of the right atrioventricular valve. In the study of the atrioventricular connection, the absent valve is substituted by a dense and refringent band, in part composed of fat (sulcus tissue), being necessary to take various slices to demonstrate that it extends to the center of the heart, and there is no tricuspid valve, neither an hypoplastic one. A false positive diagnosis of tricuspid atresia may be done if only an axial slice is evaluated, which may foreshorten the view of the right ventricle. CMR is also superior to echocardiography to evaluate potential candidates for surgical atrio-pulmonary o cavo-pulmonary connexion (Fontan-type circulationr) as it usually gives a more complete information about the morphology and size of the pulmonary arteries, data which are essential for the prognosis.[42, 43]

In patients who have undergone a Fontan-type operation (systemic venous return directly entering the pulmonary arteries), CMR with spin echo or GRE can be very useful to study the atriopulmonary connection[44], o the cavo-pulmonary connection. It may help in the diagnosis of a possible obstruccion at level of the connexion, either it has been accomplished directly (Figure 8.33) or with the interposition of prosthetic material[45]. Some authors have also shown that the technique of phase velocity mapping can be of help in this issue, since it provides information about velocity and volume of the pulmonary flow.[46]

e. Single ventricle

It corresponds to an anomaly in which both atrioventricular valves or a common atrioventricular valve open principally (more than 50%) into a single ventricular chamber. Another rudimentary ventricular cavity also exists that may have only a trabecular component, lacking from atrioventricular and ventriculoarterial connection, called "trabeculated pouch", or may be composed of a trabecular component and an outlet tract with ventriculoarterial connection, and then is named "outlet chamber." In any case, this rudimentary cavity does not have an atrioventricular

inlet component, and, therefore, does not constitute a true ventricle. There are different types of single ventricle, depending on its morphology, atrioventricular and ventriculoarterial connections. Depending on their morphology there can be: 1) right-type single ventricle; 2) left-type single ventricle, or 3) indeterminate-type single ventricle, lacking of rudimentary chamber. They may have different types o modes of atrioventricular connection: by two valves, by a single valve; one of the valves may be absent; the valves can be hypoplastic or insufficient or they can be in a straddling or overriding position. Ventriculoarterial connection can be of the different types: concordant, discordant or "double outlet," etc, and pulmonary stenosis or atresia may exist. The most typical form consists of a left-type single ventricle with two atrioventricular valves and discordant ventriculoarterial connection. The outlet chamber is located in an anterior and usually left position, although it can be placed anteriorly and to the right or directly anterior. The aorta that arises from the outlet chamber is usually located in a position anterior and to the left of the pulmonary artery. When the ventriculoarterial connection is concordant, the pulmonary artery is situated anterior and to the left of the aorta. In some cases they can be placed side by side. In the right-type single ventricle, the rudimentary chamber is situated in a posterior position and, since the ventriculoarterial connection is usually of a "double outlet" type, it is normally small, composed only of the trabecular portion (trabeculated pouch). The double inlet atrioventricular connection, the presence of one or two atrioventricular valves (Figure 8.34), the morphology and trabeculation of the single ventricle, the position of the rudimentary chamber, the position of the interventricular septum and the presence, size and location of the bulboventricular foramen may be displayed by using the SE CMR technique with axial or four-chamber slices. This allows not only the diagnosis of the single ventricle but also to classify its and to detect some possible associated anomalies.[47] Sagittal (Figure 8.35) and coronal (Figure 8.36) slices are of great utility, especially for the study of the ventriculoarterial connection as well as for the position of the great vessels. The GRE technique may confirm the diagnosis as it depicts the flow from both atria entering in a single ventricle cavity through the atrioventricular valvular floor. Likewise, it permits to evaluate the existence of possible valvular regurgitations.

f. Double outlet right ventricle

As the name indicates, in this type of anomaly, the two great vessels (aorta and pulmonary artery) arise from the right ventricle. Blood from the left ventricle drains into the right ventricle, through a ventricular septal defect that can be placed at subaortic, or subpulmonic position (Taussig-Bing), at the level of the inlet septum, or, separated from any valvular structure, at level of the muscular septum, this point being important with respect to surgical possibilities and results. The clinical manifestations basically depend on the size of the ventricular septal defect and on the presence or absence of an associated pulmonic stenosis. In cases of a large ventricular septal defect, without obstruction to the pulmonary flow, the symptoms are those of an important lef-to-right shunt (except when it is associated with pulmonary arterial vasculopathy). When there is a significant pulmonic stenosis, the clinical picture mimics a case of tetralogy of Fallot. The size of the ventricular septal defect is an important point. In cases of restrictive defects (muscular defects have a tendency to diminish in size) the blood flow to the systemic circuit and that from the pulmonary circuit will be obstructed.

As has been previously mentioned, the type of surgery and its results will basically depend on the relationship among the great vessels, the interventricular septal defect and the tricuspid valve, as well as on the associated anomalies, especially ventricular hypoplasia, ventricular cavities in superior-inferior position, stenosis of pulmonary outflow tract or anomalies of the atrioventricular valves. CMR allows to display both great vessels arising from the right ventricle, and to study the morphology of the infundibular septum, by using axial slices at different levels and with the help of sagittal and coronal slices (occasionally with a certain obliquity), it permits to localize and quantify the size of the ventricular septal defect,[48] to determine the position and dimensions of the ventricular chambers, to study the outflow tracts and to determine the relative position of the great vessels. When the ventricular septal defect is subaortic, the aorta is usually in a posterior position and to the right (occasionally "side by side" and to the right) of the pulmonary artery. When the defect is subpulmonary, the aorta is usually in an anterior position and to the right of the pulmonary artery (Figure 8.37). Cine CMR can be helpful in the diagnosis of an associated pulmonic stenosis.

8.12 Postoperative Studies

Surgical treatment of congenital heart disease has greatly evolved during the last few years, and it has changed the survival rate of those patients suffering from complex congenital anomalies. A new population composed of adolescents or adults with complex congenital heart disease has emerged. A great amount of these patients have been submitted to a type of surgery named "corrective", although rarely "curative". These patients usually present some residual lesions o sequelas from surgery, that require subsequent control. It is in these cases that CMR, without limitations concerning to acoustic window and with a wide field of view, demonstrates its greatest utility. In this section we will concentrate on a few palliative techniques, such as surgical shunts and on pulmonary banding, since some corrective techniques have already been described in previous sections.

a. Surgical arteriovenous fistulas

The surgical performance of an arteriovenous shunt in order to increase pulmonary flow was the first surgical technique employed in patients with cyanotic congenital heart disease. Different types of fistulas do exist, depending on the vessels used. The fistula of Blalock-Taussig consists in a termino-lateral anastomosis between the subclavian artery and the pulmonary artery on the same side. When this connection is made with the interposition of a prosthetic conduit, it is designated as "modified Blalock-Taussig fistula". Waterston and Potts fistulas are central shunts. In the former, the ascending aorta connects with the right pulmonary artery, while in the latter it is the descending aorta which connects with the left pulmonary artery. In both cases, the

FIGURE 8.33

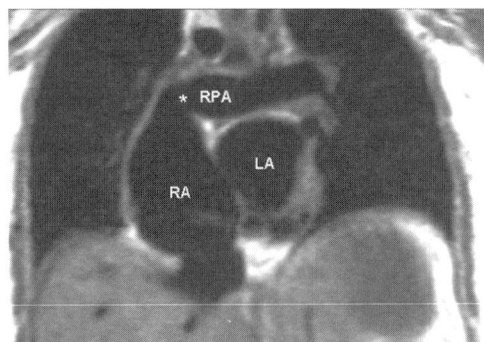

FIGURE 8.34

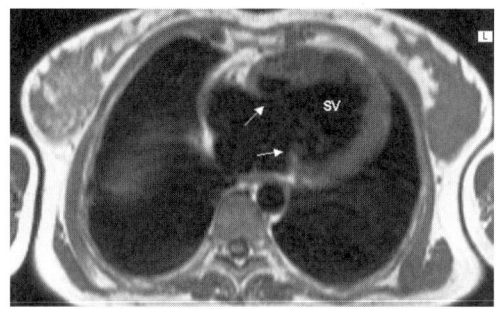

FIGURE 8.35

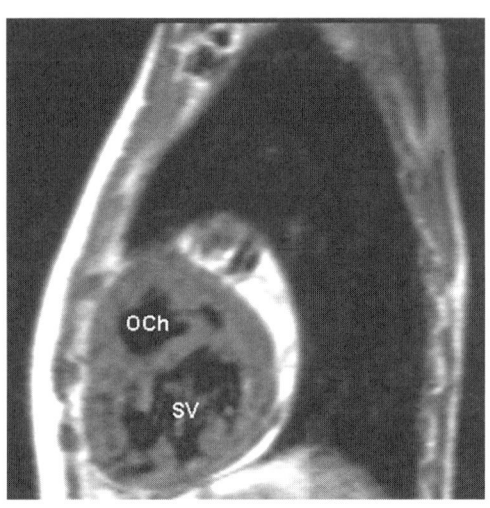

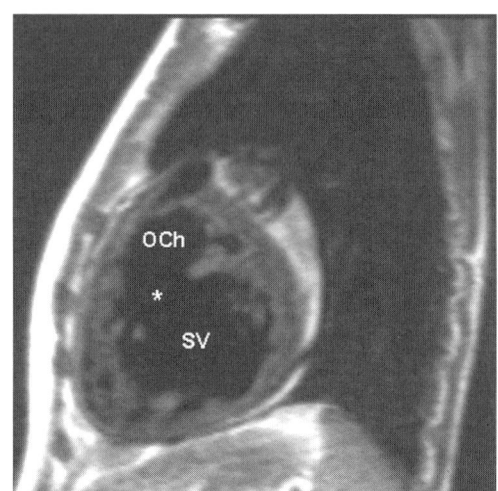

FIGURE 8.36

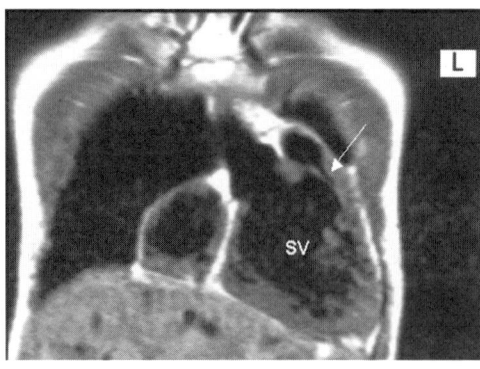

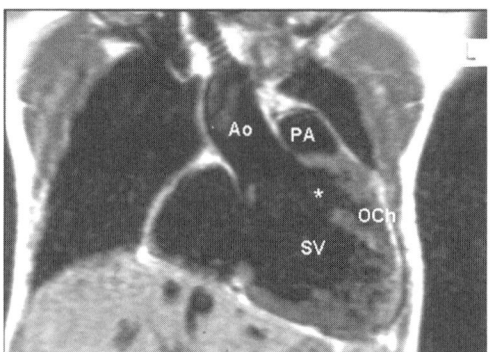

FIGURE 8.37

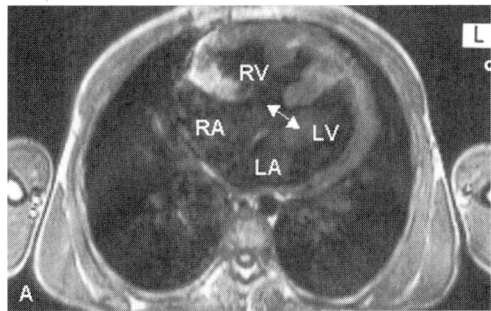 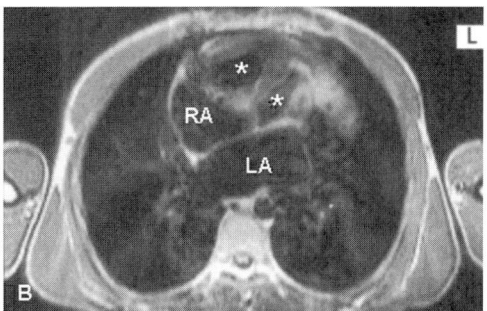

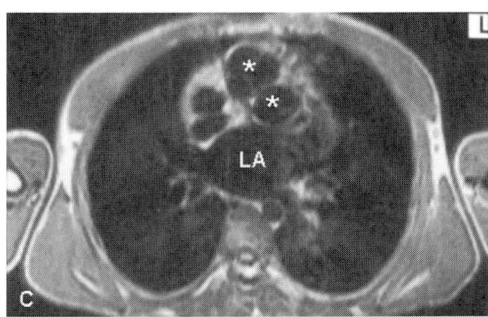 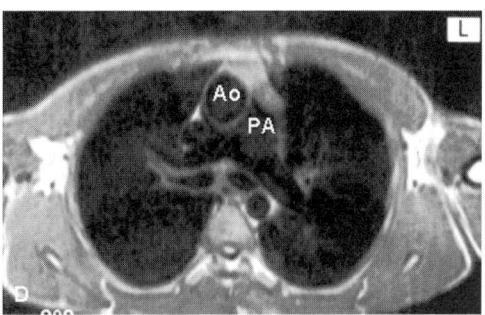

F. 8.33. Coronal T1w SE section in a patient submitted to a Fontan-type operation: the right atrium (RA) has been directly connected (asterisk) to the right pulmonary artery (RPA). LA: left atrium.

F. 8.34. Axial T1w SE plane that shows a single atrioventricular valve (arrows) in a case of single ventricle (SV) left ventricular type.

F. 8.35. Left type single ventricle (SV). Sagittal planes from left to right. Note the location of the outlet chamber (OCh) in a superior position to the single ventricle. A large bulboventricular foramen (asterisk) permits communication between both chambers.

F. 8.36. Images corresponding to the same patient than in Figure 8.34. Coronal planes from anterior (left) to posterior (right). See the outlet chamber (OCh) placed superior and to the left of the single ventricle (SV). A large bulboventricular foramen communicates both chambers (asterisk). The ventriculoarterial connection is concordant: aorta (Ao) commes off the left type single ventricle, and pulmonary artery (PA) arises from the oulet chamber. There is an associated infundibular pulmonic stenosis (arrow).

F. 8.37. Series of axial T1w SE sections in caudo-cranial order, from A to D, in a patient with a double-outlet right ventricle. A: Right (RA) and left (LA) atria are seen in a normal position; a large ventricular septal defect (arrow) communicates the right (RV) and left (LV) ventricles. B: two separate outflow chambers (asterisks) are seen emerging from the RV. C: two independent sigmoid valves (asterisks) are present, each one arising from each one of the outflow chambers. D: the great vessel arising anteriorly and to the right is the aorta (Ao), while the pulmonary artery (PA), which is identified by its bifurcation, emerges from the outlet situated posteriorly and to the left.

FIGURE 8.38

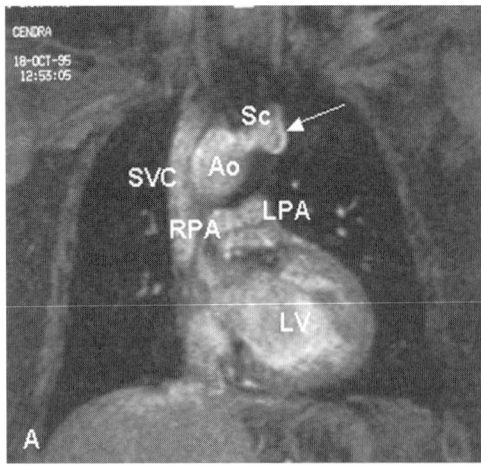
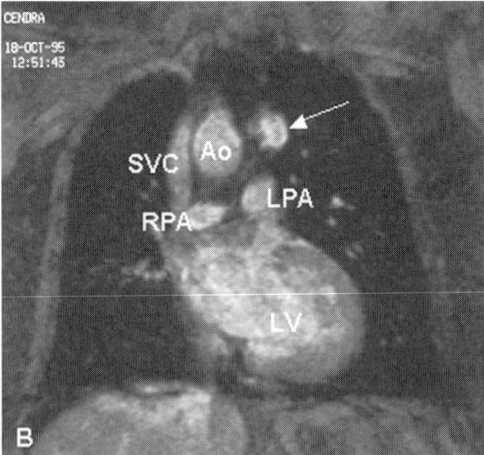
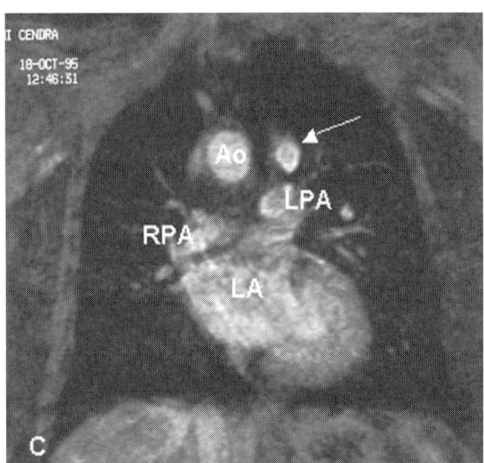
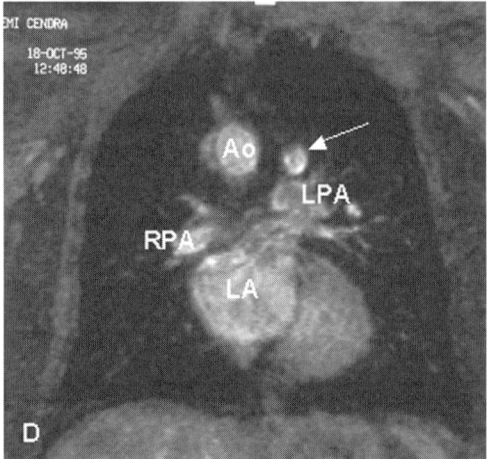

F. 8.38. Fast segmented GRE coronal planes on an anterior-posterior order, from A to D, in a patient with tetralogy of Fallot and a Blalock-Taussig fistula (arrows). The course of the fistula is seen from its origin on the left subclavian artery (Sc) (in A) down to its distal end, on the left pulmonary artery (LPA) (in D), the high signal intensity indicating flow patency of the fistula. Ao: aorta; LA: left atrium; LV: left ventricle; RPA: right pulmonary artery; SVC: superior vena cava.

connection can be either direct or by means of prosthetic material. In the Glenn fistula, the right superior vena cava is connected to the right pulmonary artery . It may be done with (classic Glenn) or without disconnection of the right pulmonary artery from the pulmonary arterial trunk and the left pulmonary branch (bidirectional Glenn).

CMR is a highly useful technique for the morphological and functional study of surgical fistulas, due to its wide field of view and its capacity for visualizing extracardiac structures.[49] In the majority of cases, it is necessary to analyze different projections and differents section levels in order to carry out a complete study of the fistulas. Axial slices usually provide the necessary information for the study of Waterston and Potts fistulas, while sagittal and coronal slices are generally more useful for the study of Blalock-Taussig (Figure 8.38) and Glenn fistulas, which on occasion require a slight obliquity in order to obtain a better alignment of their course. By means of the SE technique and cine CMR it is possible to detect possible stenosis or distortions both of the fistula itself and of the pulmonary artery used in the anastomosis.

b. Banding of the pulmonary artery

In some types of congenital heart diseases with increased pulmonary flow, when corrective surgical treatment is not possible, the banding of the pulmonary arterial trunk with the purpose of decrease the flow throughout the pulmonary circulation may be indicated. By using axial, sagittal and coronal slices, CMR may be useful to study it, being even possible by using phase velocity mapping to calculate the gradient.[50] CMR is especially useful in those cases where the banding has migrated toward a superior portion of the pulmonary arterial trunk, and with a difficult visualization by echocardiography.

References

1. Higgins ChB, Byrd BF, Farmer DW, Osaki L, Silverman NH, Cheitlin MD. Magnetic resonance imaging in patients with congenital heart disease. Circulation 1984; 70: 851–860.

2. Chung KJ, Simpson IA, Newman R. Sahn DJ, Sherman FS, Hesselink JR. Cine magnetic resonance imaging for evaluation of congenital heart disease: role in pediatric cardiology compared with echocardiography and angiography. J Pediatr 1988; 113: 1.028–1.035.

3. Simpson IA, Sahn DJ, Chung KJ. Noninvasive evaluation of congenital heart disease: Doppler ultrasound or magnetic resonance imaging. Echocardiography 1986; 6: 125–129.

4. Didier D, Ratib O, Beghetti M, Oberhaensli I, Friedli B. Morphologic and Functional Evaluation of Congenital Heart Disease by Magnetic Resonance Imaging. J Magn Reson Imaging, 1999; 10:639–55.

5. Roest AW, Helbing WA, van der Wall EE, de Roos A. Postoperative Evaluation of Congenital Heart Disease by Magnetic Resonance Imaging. J Magn Reson Imaging, 1999; 10: 656–666.

6. Boxt LM. Magnetic Resonance And Conmputed Tomographic Evaluation of Congenital Heart Disease. J Magn Reson Imaging, 2004; 19:827–847.

7. Weinberg PM, Fogel MA. Cardiac MR imaging in congenital heart disease. Cardiol Clin 1998; 16: 315–348.

8. Hartnell GG, Cohen MC, Meier RA, Finn JP. Magnetic resonance angiography demonstration of congenital heart disease in adults. Clin Radiol 1996; 51: 851–857.

9. Hirsch R, Kilner PJ, Conelly MS, Redington AN, St John Sutton MG, Sommerville J. Diagnosis in adolescents and adults with congenital heart disease. Prospective assessment of individual and combined roles of magnetic resonance imaging and transesophageal echocardiography. Circulation 1994; 90: 2.937–2.951.

10. Boothroyd A. Magnetic resonance—its current and future role in paediatric cardiac radiology. Eur J Radiol. 1998; 26: 154–62.

11. Kersting-Sommerhoff BA, Diethelm L, Stanger P, Dery R, Higashino SM, Higgins SS, Higgins CB. Evaluation of complex congenital ventricular anomalies with magnetic resonance imaging. Am HeartJ 1990; 120: 133–142.

12. Masui T, Seelos KC, Kersting-Sommerhoff BA, Higgins ChB. Abnormalities of the pulmonary veins: evaluation with MR imaging and comparison with cardiac angiography and echocardiography. Radiology 1991; 181: 645–649.

13. Julsrud PR, Ehman RL. The 'broken ring' sign in magnetic resonance imaging of partial anomalous pulmonary venous connection to the superior vena cava. Mayo Clin Proc 1985; 60: 874–879.

14. Wight CM, Barrat-Boyes BG, Calder AL, Neutze JM, Brandt PW. Total anomalous pulmonary venous connection: long-term results following repair in infancy. J Thorac Cardiovasc Sur 1977; 75: 52–63.

15. Katz NM, Kirklin JW, Pacifico AD. Concepts and practices in surgery for total anomalous pulmonary venous connection. Ann Thorac Surg 1978; 25: 479–487.

16. Gomes AS, Lois JF, Williams RG. Pulmonary arteries: MR imaging in patients with congenital obstruction of the right ventricular outflow tract. Radiology 1 990; 174: 51–57.

17. Rees S, Firmin D, Mohiaddin R, Underwood R, Longmore D. Application of flow measurements by magnetic resonance velocity mapping to congenital heart disease. Am J Cardiol 1989; 64: 953–956.

18. Wang ZJ, Reddy GP, Gotway MB, Yeh BM, Higgins ChB. Cardiovascular Shunts: MR Imaging Evaluation RadioGraphics 2003; 23: 181–194.

19. Diethelm L, Dery R, Lipton MJ, Higgins CB. Atrial-level shunts: sensitivity and specificity of MR diagnosis. Radiology 1987; 162: 181–186.

20. Powell AJ, Tsai-Goodman B, Prakash A, Greil GF, and Geva T. Comparison Between Phase-Velocity Cine Magnetic Resonance Imaging and Invasive Oximetry for Quantification of Atrial Shunts. Am J Cardiol, 2003; 91: 1523–5

21. Brenner LD, Caputo GR, Mostbeck G, Steiman D, Dulce M, Cheitlin MD, O'Sullivan M, Higgins CB. Quantification of left to right atrial shunts with velocity-encoded cine nuclear magnetic resonance imaging. JAm Coll Cardiol 1992; 20: 1.246–1.250.

22. Baker EJ, Ayton V, Smith MA, Parsons JM, Ladusans EJ, Anderson RH, Maisey MN, Tynan M, Fagg NK. Magnetic resonance imaging at a high field strength of ventricular septal defects in infants. Br HeartJ 1989; 62: 305–310.

23. Didier D, Higgins CB. Identification and localization of ventricular septal defect by gated magnetic resonance imaging.AmJ Cardiol 1986; 57: 1.363–1.368.

24. Parsons JM, Baker EJ, Anderson RH, Ladusans EJ, Hayes A, Qureshi SA, Deverall PB, Fagg N, Cook A, Maisey MN, et al. Morphological evaluation of atrioventricular septal defects by magnetic resonance imaging. Br Heart J. 1990.64(2):138–45

25. Wenink ACG, Ottenkamp J, Guit GL, Draulans NoeY, Doornbos J. Correlation of morphology of the left ventricular outflow tract with two-dimensional Doppler echocardiography and magnetic resonance imaging in atrioventricular septal defect. Am J Cardiol 1989; 63: 1.1371.140.

26. Chien CT, Lin CS, HsuYH, Lin MC, Chen KS, Wu DJ. Potencial diagnosis of hemodinamic abnormalities in patent ductus arteriosus by cine magnetic resonance imaging. Am Heart J 1991; 122: 1.065–1.072.

27. Schmid M, Theissen P, Deutsch HJ, Erdmann E, Schicha H. Magnetic Resonance Imaging of Ductus Arteriosus Botalli apertus in adulthood. Int J cardiol, 1999; 68:225–9.

28. Kilner PJ, Firmin DN, O'Rees RS, Martinez J, Penell DJ, Mohiaddin RH, Underwood SR, Longmore DB. Valve and great vessels stenosis: assessment with MR jet velocity mapping. Radiology 1991; 178: 229–235.

29. Markiewicz W, Sechtem U, Higgins CB. Evaluation of the right ventricle by magnetic resonance imaging. Am HeartJ 1987; 113: 8–14.

30. Wesley Vick III G, Rokey R, Huhta JC, Mulvagh SL, Johnston DL. Nuclear magnetic resonance imaging of the pulmonary arteries, subpulmonar region, and aortopulmonary shunts: a comparative study with two-dimensional echocardiography and angiography. Am Heart J 1990; 119: 1.103–1.110.

31. Baker EJ, AytonV, Smith MA, Parsons JM, Maisey MN, Ladusans EJ, Anderson RH, Tynan M, Yates AK, Deverall PB. Magnetic resonance imaging at high field strength of ventricular septal defects in infants Br HeartJ 1989; 62: 97–101.

32. Steffens JC, Bourne MW, Sakuma H, MOS, Higgins CB. Quantification of collateral blood flow in coarctation of the aorta by velocity encoded cine magnetic resonance imaging. Circulation, 1994; 90:937–43

33. Teien DE, Wendel H, Björnebrink J, Ekelund L. Evaluation of anatomical obstruction by Doppler echocardiography and magnetic resonance imaging in patients with coarctation of the aorta. Br Heart J 1993; 69: 352–355.

34. Mirowitz SA, Gutierrez FR, Canter CE,Vannier MW. Tetralogy of Fallot: MR imaging. Radiology 1989; 171: 207–212.

35. Davlouros PA, Kilner PhJ, Hornung TS, Li W, Francis JM, Moon JCC, Smith GC, Tat T, Pennell DJ, Gatzoulis MA. Right Ventricular Function in Adults With Repaired Tetralogy of fallot Assessed With Cardiovascular Magnetc Resonance Imaging: Detrimental Role of Right Ventricular Outflow Aneurysms or Akinesia and Adverse Right-to-Left Ventricuar Interaction. J Am Coll Cardiol, 2002; 40:2044–52.

36. Sechtem U, Jungehülsing M, de Vivie R, Mennicken U, Höpp HW. Left hemitruncus in adulthood: diagnostic role of magnetic resonance imaging. Eur Heart J 1991; 12: 1.040–1.044.

37. Ichida F, Hashimoto I, Tsubata S, Hamamichi Y, Uese K, Murakami A, Miyawaki T. Evaluation of pulmonary blood supply by multiplanar cine magnetic resonance imaging in patients with pulmonary atresia and severe pulmonary stenosis. Int J Card Imaging, 1999;15(6):473–81.

38. Mustard WT. Successful two-stage correction of transposition of the great vessels. Surgery 1964; 55: 469–472.

39. Senning A. Surgical correction of transposition of the great vessels. Surgery 1959; 45: 966–969.

40. Campbell RM, Moreau GA, Johns JA, Burger JD, Mazer M, Graham TP, Kulkarni MV. Detection of caval obstruction by magnetic resonance imaging after intraatrial repair of transposition of the great arteries. Am J Cardiol 1987; 60: 688–691.

41. Jatene AD, Fontes VF, Souza LCB, Paulista PPA, Abdulmassih N, Soussa JEMR. Anatomic correction of transposition of the great arteries. J Thorac Cardiovasc Surg 1982; 83: 20–26.

42. Fogel MA, Donofrio MT, Ramaciotti C, Hubbard AM, Weinberg PM. Magnetic resonance and echocardiographic imaging of pulmonary artery size throught stages of Fontan reconstruction. Circulation 1994; 90: 2.927–2.936.

43. Julsrud PR, Ehmann RL, Hagler DJ, Ilstrup DM. Extracardiac vasculature in candidate for Fontan surgery: MR imaging. Radiology 1989; 173: 503–506.

44. Canter E, Gutierrez FR, Molina P, Hartmann AF, Spray TL. Noninvasive diagnosis of right-sided extracardiac conduit obstructon by combined magnetic resonance imaging and continuous-wave Doppler echocardiography. J Thorac Cardiovasc Surg 1991; 101: 724–731.

45. Donelly LF, Strife JL, Bailey WW. Extrinsic airway compresion secondary to pulmonary arterial conduits: MR findings. Pediatr Radiol 1997; 27: 268–270.

46. Rebergen SA, Ottenkamp J, Doornbos J, van der Wall EE, Chin JGJ, de Roos A. Postoperative pulmonary flow dinamics after Fontan surgery: assessment with nuclear magnetic resonance velocity mapping. J Am Coll Cardiol 1993; 21: 123–131.

47. Huggon IC, Baker EJ, Maisey MN, Kakadekar AP, Graves P, Qureshi P, Tynan M. Magnetic resonance imaging of hearts with atrioventricular valve atresia or double inlet ventricle. Br HeartJ 1992; 68: 313–319.

48. Yoo SJ, Lim TH, Park IS, Hong CY, Song MG, Kim SH, Lee JH. MR anatomy of ventricular septal defect in double-outlet right ventricle with situs solitus and atrioventricular concordance. Radiology 1991; 181: 501505.

49. Jacobstein MD, Fletcher BD, Nelson D, Clampitt M, Alfidi RJ, Riemenschneider TA. Magnetic resonance imaging: evaluation of palliative systemic-pulmonary artery shunts. Circulation 1984; 70: 650–656.

50. Simpson IA, Valdes-Cruz LM, Berthoty DP, Powell JB, Hesslink JR, Chung KJ, Sahn DJ. Cine magnetic resonance imaging and color Doppler flow mapping in infants and childres with pulmonary artery bands. Am J Cardiol 1993; 71: 1.419–1.426.

Index